INTERPROFESSIONAL AND INTRAPROFESSIONAL TEAMWORK AND HANDOVERS IN HEALTHCARE

INTERPROFESSIONAL AND INTRAPROFESSIONAL TEAMWORK AND HANDOVERS IN HEALTHCARE

CHALLENGES AND RECOMMENDATIONS FROM WORK-BASED LEARNING

Carlo Lazzari • Carol Costley • Elda Nikolou-Walker

First published in 2024 by Libri Publishing

Copyright © Libri Publishing

The right of Carlo Lazzari, Carol Costley and Elda Nikolou-Walker to be identified as the authors of this work has been asserted in accordance with the Copyright, Designs and Patents Act, 1988.

ISBN 978-1-911451-24-2

A CIP catalogue record for this book is available from The British Library

Cover and design by Carnegie Book Production

Libri Publishing
Brunel House
Volunteer Way
Faringdon
Oxfordshire
SN7 7YR

Tel: +44 (0)845 873 3837

www.libripublishing.co.uk

*This book is dedicated to our colleagues
in the teams where we work who help us understand
the deep human value of professional collaboration.*

Contents

Preface

This book analyses a series of authors' interprofessional and interdisciplinary practice publications. It has then been developed to achieve a format suitable for the public. The retrospective analysis and the extracted studies are supplemented with theoretical insights and practical applications. The aim is to produce policy recommendations for interprofessional practice in healthcare. Although the reported research initially occurred in mental health settings and interprofessional teams, we could extrapolate its implications to all healthcare locations. Interprofessional collaboration occurs when individuals from different fields work and communicate to achieve a shared goal. Healthcare professionals in multidisciplinary practice aim to ensure high-quality and safe patient treatment and reach shared organisational goals. Using our research findings, we posit middle-range theories for practice-based applications in interprofessional teams. The book aims to discover and propose effective interprofessional procedures to appeal to policymakers. It also suggests plans for implementing better team collaboration, advancing the standard of care and patient safety, reducing health inequalities and promoting increased work satisfaction in multidisciplinary teams.

London, August 2023

List of Abbreviations

Carer = any HCP
CH = Clinical Handover
EBP = Evidence-Based Practice
HCP = Healthcare Professional. It also means any individual with
    a clinical or non-clinical role, whether a government official,
    employee, government agency representative or other public or
    private sector organisation[1].
HSCP = Health and Social Care Professional
MHP = Mental Health Professional
PBE = Practice-Based Evidence
SNA = Social Network Analysis
WBL = Work-Based Learning

---

1 Law Insider. *Definition of Healthcare Profession* [Online]. Available at: https://www.lawinsider.com/

CHAPTER 1

Introduction

Why we chose interprofessional studies

We are healthcare professionals and university teachers with healthcare policies and education expertise. As explored in the following chapters, we became interested in team dynamics and practice when working in hospitals or studying interdisciplinary healthcare and education. Several aspects of interdisciplinary and interprofessional teamwork appeared as the lever for patient improvement, quality of care, team coordination, and work satisfaction. In practice and education, *interprofessional cooperation* is the meeting, interacting, learning, communicating and practising of people from two or more different professional backgrounds with the customer as the care centre (Prentice et al., 2015). Additionally, reciprocal communication and comprehension of each professional's role are believed to lead to better care coordination (Prentice et al., 2015).

As we proceeded in our study, our observations gradually matured, and we began focusing our research on healthcare teams in public and private hospitals and healthcare settings where we worked or researched. This book demonstrates how we applied our learning experiences to such groups. Even from our early practice in hospitals and healthcare settings, we have observed that only integrated and interprofessional teams can deliver an adequate quality of care to patients. These last also are part of the interprofessional network, which addresses patients' needs, and it would be an error not to consider them as such.

However, patients could still be at risk of receiving less-than-optimal care from such teams, owing to the possibility of reduced information sharing and knowledge management within such teams, organisations and carers. Similarly, service users might be unwilling to disclose personal details and symptoms to carers with fears of reduced care, reluctance to being discharged from the hospital, or hope that maintaining a high profile in the severity of symptoms might attract more intensive care (Lazzari, Shoka and Rabottini, 2023). Yet, better follow-up and support of patients' multiple needs can only occur when interprofessional teams share information and leadership with all their members. Similarly, we also found that work satisfaction and climate were better in teams with factual collaboration between their members. Moreover, the safety and health of each practitioner were superior in those teams where clinical information was freely circulated, and such shared knowledge resulted in improved clinical practice (Figure 1.1).

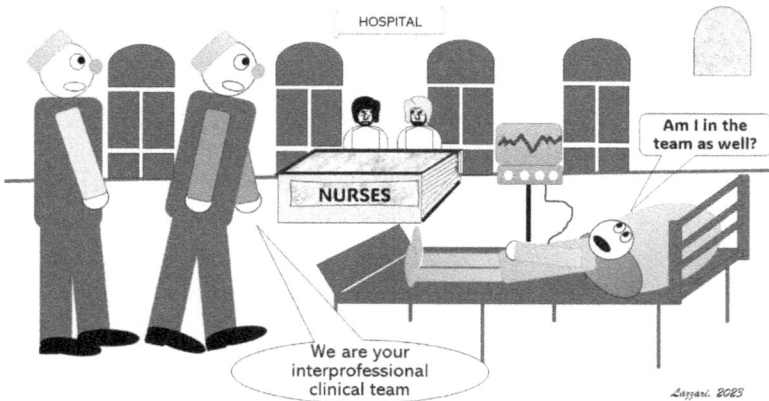

Figure 1.1. – Patients, too, are part and participants of interprofessional teams.

This book demonstrates how we applied our personal and qualified experiences to understand interprofessional practice and offer better patient care and a collaborative approach. We collaborated with highly skilled groups of practitioners. This interprofessional training enhanced our understanding of the actions needed to act synergically and acknowledge individual members' skills in pursuing common goals. In this chapter, we will inspect the terms and meanings of interprofessional practice, our learning pathway and the lessons we learned, analysed and reported in the eight chapters of this book.

Regarding the chosen publications that support each chapter, some others were not extensively included in the book due to the selection limitations to only significant publications, the partial impact factor of the journals in which other articles were published or their narrow methodological strength. We know this aspect might have increased the selection bias in our reporting. Although there has been a collection of some seminal studies, we are aware that the detailed analysis of other manuscripts with theoretical and practical applications might have added extra value or meaning to this current book (see Ioannidis et al., 2014). Furthermore, as the implication of the selected studies might threaten the transferability and generalisability of the findings, we aimed to maintain and reinforce the clinical validity of our observations throughout the book. One way to go in this direction was to extract the middle-range theories (MRTs)[1] that possibly allow inferences to be applied to other contexts and realities (see Ferguson, 2004).

In this manuscript, we narrate our professional experiences and critique our published works. In doing so, we endeavour to be analytic in our reflection, spontaneous in exploring our experience and transparent in our feelings associated with our expertise while processing them. Moreover, wherever possible, we aimed to challenge our assumptions (Bassot, 2016). When choosing a research topic, we sought one that contributed to a professional context to which we felt inclined to donate and had scholarly merit (Costley et al., 2010). Practitioner-led and practice-based research allowed us to participate directly in the research process and communicate our findings to the relevant community with increased credibility (Costley and Fulton, 2018). Schön (1987), arguing that the technical rationality paradigm is insufficient to describe the practice, proposes an epistemology of training that identifies knowledge

---

1 Robert K. Merton coined the term 'middle-range theory' in the late 1940s to bridge the gap between abstract social theory and real-world phenomena. [Ref. Oxford Reference (2023) *Middle range theory*. [Online] Available at: https://www.oxfordreference.com].

in the practical ability and creativity that certain practitioners bring to various professional contexts (Kinsella, 2009). Variability, unpredictability, originality and value conflict are all characteristics of practice, according to Schön, and here is where the core aspects of training are debated (Kinsella, 2009). An essential element of our research interest was evidence, demonstrating that ineffective interprofessional teams can lead to harmful practice and, in some cases, to professional negligence.

According to the Royal College of Physicians, the most common cause of allegations of professional negligence is a failure to effectively cooperate and share information within interprofessional teams (Germain, 2001). Several professional organisations endorse collaborative practice within teams.

General Medical Council's (GMC, 2022a) *Code of Practice*, which regulates UK doctors, offers guidelines for teamwork, suggesting that (1) doctors must appreciate the abilities and contributions of their colleagues while collaborating with them, (2) they must treat co-workers with fairness and decency, and (3) doctors must be conscious of how their behaviour affects others within and outside the team.

The Nurse and Midwifery Council's (2015) *Code* suggests that to work collaboratively with colleagues and to maintain the safety of those receiving care, nurses and other allied professionals should apply effective communication with one another, respect the skills, knowledge, and contributions of their co-workers, refer issues to them when necessary, and share information to find and minimise risks.

The British Psychological Society's (2017) *Practice Guideline* suggests that in a number of the fields where psychologists work, national policy and legislation mandate collaboration and cooperation with colleagues for the benefit of clients, the advancement of safety and protection of the general public, or the organisation itself.

The Royal College of Surgeons of England's (2022) *Professional Code of Conduct* suggests that to work collaboratively, surgeons should communicate effectively with other team members while being open to their feedback and keenly reflecting on it when focusing on practice and conduct.

The Royal College of Psychiatrists (2019) *Working Together* policy paper suggests that collaborative practice is when mental health practitioners respect and maximise the knowledge and capabilities of co-workers, service users and their family or friends while reducing hierarchies and fostering respect; collaborative practice allows anyone in a team to contribute equally to decision-making; cooperative procedures also consent group learning through mindfulness of interpersonal mistakes and achievements.

The Royal College of Nursing in the UK (2022), regulating UK nurses advises that (1) teams are a need in the workplace; (2) the health of a team or teams influences the safety of patients; (3) the performance of a team may be affected by its size, composition and internal dynamics, as well as by its leadership style; (4) teamwork includes team structures and procedures; (5) the structure is associated not just with size, responsibilities and hierarchical type but also to recognised modes of conduct and (6) any of these may have an impact on team cohesiveness.

The British Psychological Society (BPS, 2017), which regulates the activities of UK psychologists, emphasises the role of leadership in teams and maintains that leadership is often cited and defined through the framework that leading change is to accept the responsibility of creating circumstances that allow people to accomplish a common objective despite uncertainties; in general, contemporary leadership approaches are better connected with team or system work.

The College of Social Workers (Thomas and Baron, 2012) suggests that practical interprofessional cooperation is a crucial constituent of successful social workers; they must successfully interact with other professionals with different areas of expertise to achieve the desired results in their work with service users and carers.

An inadequate interprofessional practice was instead found to be the root cause of unsatisfactory patient care in seventy per cent of the cases; in comparison, rigid hierarchical leadership was found to be the root cause in fifty-seven per cent of the cases, according to a review that analysed thirty studies that evaluated the obstacles to quality care in various countries (Jones and Jones, 2010). Additionally, hierarchies within healthcare teams are seen as a barrier to accessible communication within a team (Montreuil and Carnevale, 2010). Despite a wealth of research on interprofessional practice, there still appear to be gaps in the applicative part. The findings of interprofessional studies conducted in global research settings were not considered generalisable, thus reducing the validity of all research on this topic (Reeves et al., 2017). In light of this, we wanted to take a further step forward in our interprofessional study and use our public works and direct experience in the field to dig into social concepts and think inductively to generate theories of practice, thus increasing the transferability and generalisability of our findings.

According to the NHS Health Research Authority (2022), scientific enquiry should improve the evidence base, reduce uncertainties, improve care and develop staff's health and social care skills. Based on our evidence-based and practice-based research outcomes, this book aims to establish convincing evidence from our reflective practice in interprofessional teams. This process has further developed middle-range theories (MRTs), here discussed, aiming to promote a level of (inter)professionalism practice that policymakers can officially accept.

Background information and definition of terms

Each healthcare professional (HCP) abides by its regulatory organisation regarding interprofessional teamwork. To supply high-quality and safe patient care, healthcare practitioners must effectively cooperate with staff members from other health and social care disciplines inside and outside teams and organisations (GMC, 2022). Regardless of each person's area of expertise, healthcare professionals must accept and acknowledge the talents and contributions of everyone on their teams (GMC, 2022). HCPs should also inspire other team members to cooperate effectively with other teams or colleagues as well as with one another (GMC, 2022). It is important to act accordingly to deal with the difficulties that arise due to poor communication or unclear roles within or across team members, as these problems may affect patient care and safety (GMC, 2022). One of the significant tools for interprofessional collaboration and communication is clinical handover.

Clinical handover (CH) is the short- or long-term transfer of a professional's liability, information about a patient, and duty for some or all parts of a patient's care to another person or group of experts (Eggins and Slade, 2015). Handovers commonly rely on the SBAR algorithm's communication of patients' data among team members, which consists of *situations*, *backgrounds*, *assessments* and *recommendations* about a patient under examination (Eggins and Slade, 2015). According to estimations, there are over three hundred million handovers annually in the United States, more than forty million in Australia, and more than one hundred million in England, making handover undoubtedly the most significant and consistent clinical communication process in the delivery of patient care (Eggins and Slade, 2015). From the results of a recent in-depth investigation by the European Commission, failures in communication between healthcare providers are responsible for between twenty-five and forty per cent of adverse outcomes in patient care, twenty-seven per cent of instances of malpractice lawsuits and more than seventy per cent of severe clinical incidences (Eggins and Slade, 2015). Studies show that inadequate communication between nurses and physicians doubles patient mortality and lengthens hospital stays (Dingley et al., 2008). Conflicting personalities, lack of trust, disorganisation and organisational divisions have all been identified as interpersonal issues that impede relationships and interactions (Foronda, MacWilliams and McArthur, 2016).

Interprofessional communication, in the sense that it is intended to be understood by this book, refers to any practice in which two or more healthcare professionals (HCPs) working in the same or distinct teams communicate verbally and in writing to transfer information, data, observations, and duties for the assessment and treatment of communal patients who are actual service users or have been referred that team (Lazzari and Masiello, 2016). This communication or handover may happen between teams or within the same team. Communication can be synchronous, face-to-face or via telephone. However, it can also be asynchronous when written records, electronic notes, text messages, and interactions occur at different times among HCPs (Lazzari and Masiello, 2016).

For high-quality and risk-free patient care, practitioners in the healthcare industry must collaborate with their peers in other health and social care professions (GMC, 2022). Collaboration between professionals from diverse disciplines occurs when people from different fields work together to attain a common objective (Barr et al., 2016). Members of interprofessional teams have various communication skills, including verbal, written, electronic, digital or analogic, to exchange information and participate in group activities and decisions (Barr et al., 2016).

Interprofessional practice (IPP) enhances teamwork and care quality (Reeves, 2003; Reeves et al., 2011). IPP involves healthcare professionals from a variety of backgrounds working together to accomplish two goals: (1) to advance teamwork and customer care by employing effective handover, sharing decision-making, collaborating synergistically and acknowledging colleagues' knowledge, and (2) to provide collaborative care to patients, families and caregivers (Barr et al., 2008; Bridges et al., 2011; World Health Organization [WHO], 2010). Interprofessional practice in the healthcare sector may include interventions such as patient assessments, checkups, consultations, reviews, reports, paperwork, messaging services and care pathways (Reeves et al., 2011). Interprofessional cooperation is a procedure that incorporates discussion and decision-making and enhances the care given to patients or customers of an organisation (Way et al., 2000).

IPP occurs when individuals with experience in several fields collaborate effectively to accomplish a shared objective (Barr et al., 2016; Reeves, 2013). Interprofessional team members utilise communication skills (such as oral, written and electronic) and any other means of information sharing that makes it possible for all team members to partake in the collective decisions and strengthen their agreed-upon actions in the direction of a joint plan (Lazzari and Rabottini, 2021). Interprofessional teams might also be interdisciplinary (involving two or more subjects or areas of expertise)[2] teams (e.g., health carers, police officers, community organisations, and so on) (Barr et al., 2016). Interprofessional practice improves the standard of care, patient safety, and work satisfaction experienced by team members when they believe that their contributions are being considered (Thistlethwaite, Moran and WHO Study Group on Interprofessional Education and Collaborative Practice, 2010).

Regardless of whether the team members' professional backgrounds are the same or different, they can exchange vital information and data

---

2 Cambridge Dictionary Online (2023). *Definition of Interdisciplinary.* Available at: https://dictionary.cambridge.org/dictionary/english/interdisciplinary

with each other and agree on strategies to employ if they rely on each other and depend on each other's sustenance and expertise to attain their everyday goals (Barr et al., 2016). Each member of an interprofessional team should thus appreciate the importance of other members' roles in achieving communal expected goals (Barr et al., 2016).

Interprofessional education (IPE) in medicine occurs when learners from various healthcare professions (e.g., student nurses, medical students, occupational therapy students, pharmacy nurses) learn to work together towards a shared objective, such as offering a particular intervention in patient care and thus learn to appreciate the support of their colleagues with a different area of expertise (Frenk et al., 2010). The patient care benefits gained by training healthcare personnel in interprofessional care have been confirmed by a meta-analysis (Reeves et al., 2013).

Interprofessional team members share some fundamental characteristics: (1) they work with colleagues with different areas of expertise and use them as resources; (2) they engage in jargon-free communication, enabling each member to understand others easily; (3) they coordinate their efforts with those of others and work together towards a common goal; (4) they reflect on how they are perceived by other team members and use their interactions to improve collaboration, and (5) they are moved by their sincere intentions of reciprocal esteem and appreciation of other team members and their professional roles (Thistlethwaite, 2012; Thistlethwaite, Moran and WHO Study Group on Interprofessional Education and Collaborative Practice, 2010). An atmosphere of reciprocal esteem can be created in interprofessional teams by reducing general stereotypes (Thistlethwaite, Moran and WHO Study Group on Interprofessional Education and Collaborative Practice, 2010). Doing so can improve care outcomes in healthcare services (Curran et al., 2012).

Summary of key points from the frameworks

A team is a group of persons who collaborate toward a communal objective (Lynas and NHS Leadership Academy, n/d). It is hypothesised that the combined inter- and intraprofessional cooperation, particularly in patients and service users with numerous health issues, enhances the quality of their treatment (de Gans et al., 2022).

Interprofessional competencies have been divided into six areas; each one contains the significant proficiencies that team members should master to succeed in cooperative practice, (1) *teamwork* means cooperating with co-workers in related or unrelated healthcare disciplines while identifying obstacles to collaboration; (2) *roles and responsibilities* entails recognising the duties and responsibilities of each affiliate of the interprofessional unit, supplying integrated care to patients and challenging roles-related stereotypes; (3) *communication* implies sharing personal viewpoints with group members, listening intently to other participants and distributing information about shared patients effectively; (4) *critical reflection and education* aims to enhance cooperative care via self-reflective practice; (5) *interactions with patients* requires using collaborative practice to improve treatment results, client safety and reduce medical errors; and (6) *ethical performance* occurs by recognising one's own prejudices and respecting other people's viewpoints while fostering a culture of shared respect and communal values (Walsh et al., 2004; GMC, 2009; WHO, 2010; Brewer and Jones, 2013; IPEC, 2016; Lazzari, 2019).

Collaborative practice and definition of terms
Other definitions collected from several sources are the following (Reeves and Lewin, 2004; Reeves, Lewin, Espin and Zwarenstein, 2010; Jelley, Larocque and Borghese, 2013; Reeves, Xyrichis and Zwarenstein, 2018; Farlex Free Dictionary, 2023):

-interdisciplinary teamwork refers to the strategic partnerships carried out by experts from several fields, including computer science, anthropology, economics, geography, and psychology;

-interprofessional collaboration involves affiliates in health and social care professions (HSCPs) who ordinarily collaborate to resolve issues or provide solutions; whereas the integration and sense of togetherness are less critical in cooperative groups than in teams, teamwork is similar to collaboration in that both require shared accountability, some interconnectedness, and role clarity; teamwork tasks are less demanding, intricate, and unpredictable;

-**interprofessional coordination,** like cooperation, combines the efforts of affiliates in HSCPs; it is a softer working structure with less interdisciplinary contact and debate; interprofessional practice with shared identity is comparable to cooperation, although integration and dependency are less crucial; teamwork is even less urgent, complicated, and predictable than cooperation; coordination, like cooperation, involves shared responsibility and clarity of roles, duties and objectives;

-**interprofessional education** implies affiliates or apprentices of two or more HSCPs experimenting with how to cooperate to enhance teamwork and care;

-**interprofessional interventions** include members of HSCPs training and cooperating to improve outcomes;

-**interprofessional networks** are loose coalition teams of people from many HSCPs that collaborate and meet regularly; interprofessional networks are ones in which teamwork is prioritised above common team identity, positions, objectives, transparency, dependency, integration, and shared responsibility; additionally, jobs in networks are seen as predictable, uncomplicated, and non-urgent; as a consequence, networks may be virtual, with members communicating asynchronously through email or online video/audio conferencing rather than meeting in person

-**interprofessional teamwork** entails clarity, interdependence, integration, and shared responsibility; team duties in this structure are typically unexpected, urgent, and challenging; it is a type of work in which individuals from various HSCPs share team characteristics and work together in a united and interdependent manner to solve problems and provide services;

-**intraprofessional or intradisciplinary practice** has members in the same field or profession (such as nurses, physicians, and social workers) who may have various levels of education and practice scopes;

-**multidisciplinary teamwork** is teams where affiliates are drawn from several academic branches, such as psychology, sociology, and mathematics, organisations and professions instead of numerous occupations, such as medicine, nursing, and social work, who cooperate to improve their non-overlapping contributions to enhance patient care;

-**interdisciplinary** teams are founded on healthcare experts from many professions who proficiently collaborate to achieve a shared objective for patients;

-**transdisciplinary** team is a group of individuals from several fields who work together to improve patient care via practice or research (Figure 1.2.).

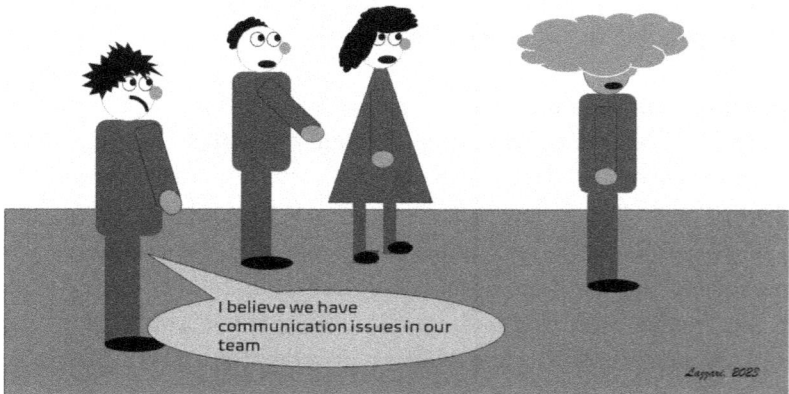

Figure 1.2. – Those who cause communication impasses in interprofessional teams might not be aware of them.

Bottlenecks in collaborative practice

As described in the current book, a *bottleneck* in collaborative care is any *block or jam* deriving from a lack of bridging communication, handovers, and duties in intra- and interprofessional teams. Although health professionals from other disciplines sometimes speak with one another, most interactions are those from the same area of speciality, which, if unhelpful, have been found conducive to medical errors in transferring information and care between professionals (Manias et al., 2021). As discussed earlier, there are risks of malpractice and patient casualties when there is less-than-optimal interprofessional practice. As highlighted by the research, bottlenecks in interprofessional communication and interaction and patient handover can result in adverse clinical events (Eggins and Slade, 2015).

For example, by crossing the *areas of expertise* and the *level of seniority experience,* we have found four possible blockages if interactions, knowledge management and information sharing rely exclusively on the following categories:

A) **intraprofessional bottlenecks** occur in unidisciplinary teams, where professionals with the same qualification (e.g., nurse-to-nurse, doctor-to-doctor, and so on) do not share information, accountability and care plans about their communal patient with colleagues from other professions:

- *interactions at the same level of seniority/expertise and same professional category* (e.g., a high-ranking nurse with a high-ranking nurse); this pattern excludes inputs from most junior or low-ranking members who might have more information about patients and more frequent contact with them (e.g., junior nurse or doctor) (Lazzari and Masiello, 2017b; Lazzari and Thomas, 2018a; Lazzari, Kotera and Thomas, 2019);
- *interactions at different levels of seniority/expertise and the same professional category* (e.g., high-ranking and student nurse); this pattern excludes inputs from other professional classes with loss of information in patient assessment and care (Lazzari, McAleer, Nusair and Rabottini, 2022);

B) **interprofessional bottlenecks** occur when professionals in multidisciplinary teams do not share information, care plans and accountability about communal patients under their care by also selecting colleagues with different qualifications or areas of seniority/expertise:

- *interactions at the same level of seniority/expertise and another professional category* (e.g., high-ranking ward manager and consultant);

by excluding colleagues with varying levels of seniority, there is a risk of reduced interprofessional learning and exclusion of more high-ranking or junior participants in decision-making (Lazzari, Kotera, Green and Rabottini, 2021);

- *interactions at different levels of seniority/expertise and another professional category* (e.g., ward manager with junior doctor); if this pattern does not cross seniority and professional boundaries, there is the risk of creating dyads or triads of people who develop hubs and close ties with the chance of biased decisions in patient care (Lazzari, McAleer, Nusair and Rabottini, 2021; Figures 1.3. and 1.4.)[3].

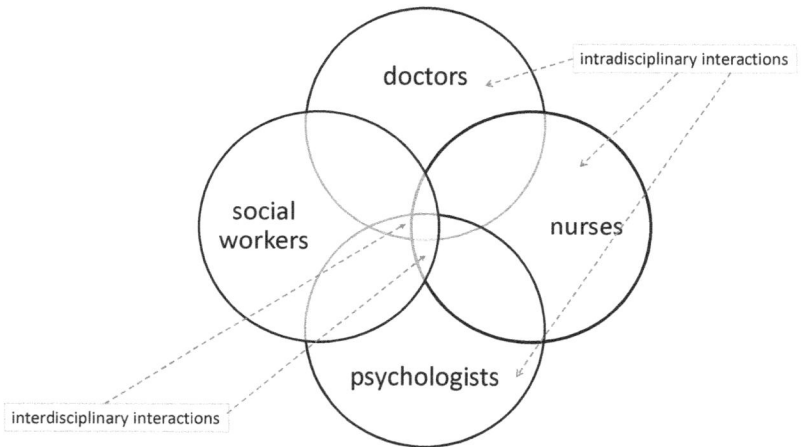

Figure 1.3. – Areas of inter- and intradisciplinary practice.

---

3 Hub is the centre of activity or focal point (Reference: Merriam-webster. com. (2019). Definition of HUB. [online] Available at: https://www.merriam-webster.com/dictionary/hub.

BOTTLENECK IS LINKED TO EXCLUSIVE INTERACTIONS WITHIN THE SAME PROFESSIONAL CATEGORY	INTRAPROFESSIONAL BOTTLENECK ↑	NURSES	DOCTORS	PSYCHO-LOGISTS	SOCIAL WORKERS	SENIO-RITY LEVEL	OF SENIORITY WITHIN THE SAME LEVEL	BOTTLENECK IS LINKED TO EXCLUSIVE INTERACTIONS WITHIN THE SAME LEVEL
		NURSE 1	DOCTOR 1	PSYCH 1	SOCWOR 1	LEVEL 1		
		NURSE 2	DOCTOR 2	PSYCH 2	SOCWOR 2	LEVEL 2		
		NURSE 3	DOCTOR 3	PSYCH 3	SOCWOR 3	LEVEL 3		
		INTERPROFESSIONAL BOTTLENECK →						

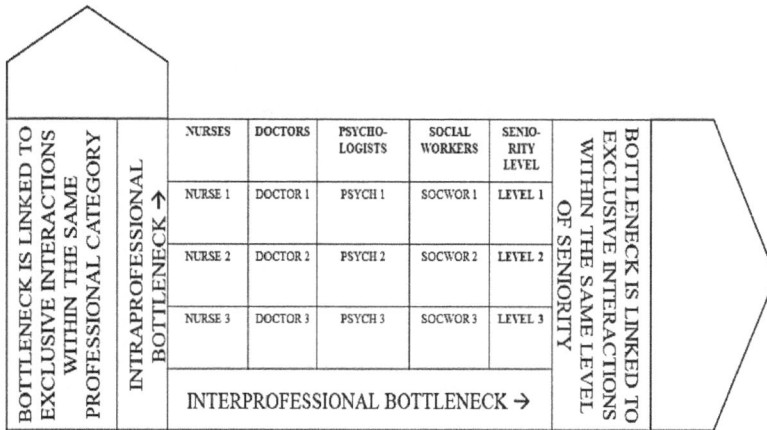

Figure 1.4. – Bottlenecks in interprofessional practice occur due to a lack of bridging in the level of seniorities or professional categories.

Developing as reflective practitioners in interprofessional practice

Interprofessional collaboration and training are central in healthcare to promote patient care, effectively communicate care plans to other practitioners, expedite patient transfer between teams and enhance a feeling of togetherness in active groups. As health and educational practitioners, interprofessional practice is one of our significant professional targets and strategies of daily work. In our professional approach, we are supervised to work in interprofessional teams. We must demonstrate to our regulatory professional bodies and employers that we can assimilate the diverse views and opinions of other healthcare professionals, patients, students and their carers or mentors while maintaining independent thought (NHS, 2022). We must also demonstrate the ability to understand and recognise the limits of our skills and determine whether to seek other professionals' views to inform our decisions (NHS, 2022).

Our interest in teamwork in healthcare and education, specifically in interprofessional practice, was triggered by our aim of improving the collaboration between team members and helping them understand how their team affiliates, with their experience and knowledge, can be resources for the whole team (see Finch, 2000). A collaborative and interprofessional practice also entails flexibility by cross-covering other roles and responsibilities, which expedites the solution of problems and work-based learning (WBL), such as when junior nurses cover shifts at more high-ranking levels (Finch, 2000).

This book explores and explains how we used our reflective practice and research instruments to capture the core elements in interprofessional practice and the bottlenecks in interprofessional communication that could cause adverse clinical events and how we used our findings to propose viable solutions to advance collaborative practice, patient safety and quality of care. Although research on interprofessional practice was already present, to our knowledge, there were limited or no studies to measure the characteristics of social networks in interprofessional teams, capture interpersonal distance and choice, and use numerical methods to quantify the strength or limitations of interpersonal links. The systematic reviews scrutinising this topic only reported qualitative studies on narratives of interprofessional teams (see Aungst and Belliveau, 2015; Foronda et al., 2016; Parry et al., 2017; Etherington et al., 2019; Bok et al., 2022; Gleeson, O'Brien, O'Mahony and Byrne, 2022; Ong et al. 2021). After extensive research, all the public works we explored in the current book illustrate novel ways to tackle interprofessional practice and try to apply social network theories to these studies.

This book is based on our progressive growth in reflectively exploring the different aspects of interprofessional teamwork and education. The selected publications were generated during our clinical and teaching practice in healthcare and learning settings. According to Schön (1991), there are two forms of reflective practice: *reflection in action*, which occurs when an occurrence is happening, with the practitioner thinking about it and acting immediately to respond to it, and *reflection on action*, after a specific circumstance, but a practitioner can still gain new information and a fresh theoretical perspective from it. Argyris and Schön (1974) presented a theory of action, or 'theory-in-use', claiming that when someone understands what to do in a specific scenario to realise an expected effect, such a person knows the theory-in-use for that situation. This condition indicates that such a person understands the nature of the consequence to be sought, the proper conduct in the context to realise it and the assumptions included in the theory (Argyris and Schön, 1974). While conducting an advanced study of interprofessional teamwork, we felt that we had started to extract ideas about collaborative care that could be applied in different settings. However, a loop reflection went from the social phenomena we observed to our interpretation and analysis and back to the social phenomenon to look for confirmation.

During this reflective loop, we used autoethnography to ponder on an issue before it became a research question, writing in the first (plural) person, breaching the conventional separation of the researcher and the topic of the investigation with inductive theories across the discussed cases (see Belbase, Luitel and Taylor, 2013). *Autoethnography* is an autobiographical category of writing for academia that draws from, analyses, or interprets the authors' personal experiences and links research findings to self-identity, cultural norms and resources, communication practices, customs, assumptions, representations, standards, shared purposes, feelings principles, and more significant problems in society, culture, and politics (Poulos, 2021).

Metamorphosis can occur using an autoethnographic approach: we transformed our perceptions and experiences of the past to inform our present and shape our future (Custer, 2014) through research. Lived experiences may frequently give insight into societal and practice-based challenges for enhanced understanding and informed decision-making when using self-inquiry research methodologies (Lewis and Thorne, 2021).

Hence, to conduct a social investigation and act as autoethnographers, we used our research material, informed by our memories of the research settings and populations, and merged the diaries we constructed before, during and after the research, including our self-reflective and self-observational notes (Chang, 2013). Before we developed a research approach, we examined our experiences through new perspectives. We sought to find and fill a 'gap' in the existing related storylines. Our autoethnography grew aesthetic and evocative, filled with stories, characters and scenes from our daily experiences (Ellis, Adams and Bochner, 2011).

Sometimes, the setting was the same as a hospital ward, a learning centre, or a medical ambulatory. Other times, different locations were scrutinised, but they were in the same healthcare speciality, usually general adult psychiatry or dementia wards, liaison psychiatric teams, community mental health, and so on. It has been reported that a few months spent in the field with meticulously detailed field notes are recommended to establish 'credibility' about the observed situation and to describe the setting and the people vividly and convincingly (Saldaña, 2011). An ethnographer's ambition is to gain a comprehensive understanding of a culture's emic perspective—that is, the way a culture's members view the world; at the same time, the aim is to acquire tacit knowledge, which is information about a culture that is so deeply embedded in the cultural experience that people do not even think about it (Polit and Beck, 2022)[4]. The description of social networks in interprofessional teams that permeates our research is somewhat an attempt to describe a healthcare culture by studying its observable behaviours and interpersonal choices.

Our motivation to progress to higher levels of Perry's (1970) cognitive and moral development also sustained the *axiological or ethical momentum* to write self-reflectively on interprofessional practice. Crafting a self-reflective book, we felt, drove us away from the dualistic perceptions of the research outcomes as representing an objective or actual reality; the *multiplicity stage* was approached by using divergent thinking and by generating hypotheses of application for findings in different social and healthcare settings; the *relativistic stage* was reached when we started to extract from the public works generalisable arguments as relative to the premises of the research debated; in the *commitment stage*, we felt we had the agency and ethical responsibility to propose changes in interprofessional practice; the *commitment stage*, as Perry suggests, is an affirmative experience where we constantly defined our identity and contributions to the world of science (see Perry, 1970).

---

4 Tacit knowledge is the collection of intangible, hard-to-communicate skills, insights, and understandings that persons acquire from their personal experiences. It is also referred to as experiential or know-how knowledge (Reference: Oragui, D. (2023) *What is tacit knowledge.* Helpjuice. Available at: https://helpjuice.com [Accessed 25 Aug 2023]).

Reflection in action

Reflection 'in action' was the immediate impact of teamwork on our cognition and emotions, what we learned and experienced when an event was happening, as applied to each of the eight chapters analysed in this book (see Schön and Martin, 1994). As written in our selected public works, we observed that interprofessional interactions often created bottlenecks in shared communication and skills within teams during our routine clinical practice. At times, team communication captured the centralisation of only some professionals despite all team members being essential to the shared knowledge about patient care. This aspect was registered as an 'ongoing' action. We used our research and observations of detectable social interactions to reflect on what was occurring in teams and how network analysis and exploring interpersonal choices could extract salient points in the teamwork we studied. At the same time, we used the literature to appreciate and create a framework that could help us decipher the observed human events.

Reflection on action

After each study project, we arrived at conclusions, endeavoured to reflect on our observations and checked whether they could be used to deliver a significant change in the observed practice. This process was the reflection *post-facto* or 'on action' stage. This last was the moment when we thought about how to use our research findings deductively. We aimed to draw conclusions that could practically impact interprofessional practice. The ultimate goal was to generate theories about our observed social worlds inductively. We were familiar with the settings we attended since we worked at the same or similar organisations where the studies were conducted. However, we could not say that our observations represented 'the reality'.

On the contrary, they represented only 'one reality' in the concerned settings and, at the moment, one that was true to us and our research instruments in a specific scenario, timeframe and team. Schön and Martin (1994) discussed the 'frame' of reference, which means that a theoretical viewpoint cannot be falsified; they felt there are no neutral theories or objective observers. These writers emphasised that the only way to make sense of social realities is via a personal frame of reference, a unique view of how social events play out (Schon and Martin, 1994). The holders of another theoretical frame of reference can interpret the same social data differently from the initial researcher (Schön and Martin, 1994).

Reflective practice

Interpreting social phenomena involves both reflexivity and reflective practice. *Reflexivity* is the ability to consider our influence on what we see in the world and how we interpret it (Fook, 2018). Being reflexive also means recognising how we and our context determine what knowledge is favoured and how it is understood to lead to better research (Fook, 2018). We are healthcare practitioners and university teachers who have grown professionally and personally in different social settings, such as hospitals, communities, universities, non-profit organisations and charities. We achieved our collective goals by integrating our efforts and skills with others. Mutual respect and empathy have always been the leitmotif or rules of engagement in our teams.

On the other hand, our *reflection* was initiated by excavating and scrutinising deeply held assumptions in our experiences to reconstruct the value of such experiences and redevelop new directives (more aligned with the healthcare policies) for practice (Fook, 2018). This activity improved moral and sympathetic interaction with the community (Fook, 2018). We scrutinised teamwork in healthcare by reflecting on the selected publications and directly on our practice. The eight chapters in the book reviewed assumptions of interprofessional work and how we restructured the interpretation of such activity, which helped us suggest new guidelines for its implementation for stakeholders and healthcare organisations.

Reflective practice and our research-based approach attempted to foster practical wisdom where we, as professionals engaged in a workplace, researched to generate valuable knowledge and communicated the findings to the relevant community (Maxwell, 2018). This book demonstrates how our research publications built knowledge about teamwork in healthcare and offered outcomes that suggest a new way forward in interprofessional partnership and enhancing patient care.

In the subsequent chapters, we will provide a more in-depth evaluation of our research and the theoretical foundations upon which it was built. Since this is a manuscript, we aim to offer a clear picture of the selected areas by identifying their relevant and recent advances. In doing so, we will also illustrate that we keep abreast of the recent developments in the field (Costley, Elliott and Gibbs, 2010).

Our research roadmap

This book was based on our selected studies on the previously published topic in the thematic areas. Similarly, the manuscript reflects significant interprofessional practice and educational research phases. We selected only the publications accepted in the journals referenced in PubMed and Google Scholar, as well as our previous books or book chapters. Each of the chosen publications reported in the book's chapters represents the final stage of a research phase, endorsed and supported by conference presentations, posters, journal articles, peer-reviewed conference abstracts and book chapters. Each thus characterises a diversified step towards a concept, conclusion, stage or theory in interprofessional practice. This book analyses these publications in separate chapters, illustrating their theoretical framework and findings.

Furthermore, for each publication, we extracted middle-range theories that condense the practical implications of the results and how these conclusions helped and can help improve interprofessional practice. The selected public works answered several *research questions*. The chapters were grounded on seminal articles generated by our research on interprofessional teams.

In Chapter 1, the current one, we jotted down the salient points to create a frame of understanding of the interprofessional practice.

In Chapter 2, we focused on our observations by joining interprofessional teams; our perspective as team participants helped throughout our research on interprofessional practice. In this chapter, theories of social interactions are merged with network analysis to focus on the distribution of tasks between professionals in psychiatric teams. Social System theories are discussed extensively (Lazzari, 2019).

In Chapter 3, we used more structured research methods and began to describe the configuration of interprofessional groups and measure the intensity of the bonds between their members. With tangible examples, we highlight how interprofessional teams allow to promote patients' biological, physical and social personhood. We explore the concepts of unitasking and multi-tasking in interprofessional teams (Lazzari, Kotera and Thomas, 2019).

In Chapter 4, we use Social Network Analysis (SNA) for qualitative and quantitative analysis of interprofessional teams, interpersonal bonds and the intensity of teamwork collaboration. We will look at how hubs of professionals are formed in terms of the power of their partnership. We will also examine the concept of periphery and exclusion (Lazzari, Kotera, Green and Rabottini, 2021).

In Chapter 5, we will investigate the aspects of interprofessional education (IPE) and the current pedagogical theories that can be applied to implement reflective learning into IPE. We found how HCPs in IPE could learn with and from others ways of reciprocal support, empathy and mutual sustenance; they all benefitted patients' satisfaction (Lazzari, McAleer, Nusair and Rabottini, 2021).

In Chapter 6, we apply bibliometrics analysis using VosViewer to extract from the Web of Science what concepts are related to those discussed in the book, such as network, interprofessional, communication, ethnography and knowledge management. Findings suggest that to promote integrated care in interprofessional teams, managers must be mindful of communication barriers and obstacles to interactions that negatively impact patient care (Lazzari, McAleer, Nusair and Rabottini, 2022).

In Chapter 7, we look in more detail at interprofessional handover and the requirements to allow the transfer of information in interprofessional teams. Collegiate use of ISBAR handoff in groups improves reciprocal actions and reduces misunderstandings and medical errors (Lazzari, 2023).

In Chapter 8, we review the theories explored and discuss in detail the influence our manuscript has and will have on interprofessional teamwork, looking into possible changes and making suggestions for policymakers. We explain how the book's findings can be transferable in similar settings and the theories behind evidence-based practice and practice-based evidence.

To direct our summaries, we used the population, intervention and outcome (PIO) question model to guide our research pathway to explore the topics of interest (Polit and Beck, 2022). The PIO questions can be explorative of the meaning or processes of interest, an evaluation of the matter, a form of assessment or an analysis of intervention (Polit and Beck, 2022). As there is no comparison group, the *population* is interprofessional teams; the *intervention* is the evaluation of teams, the assessment of the degree of centrality of some professionals, the appraisal of interprofessional education and the review of international literature on the topic; the *outcomes* the interprofessional relations, quality of care and job satisfaction (see Melnyk and Fineout-Overholt, 2019).

Regarding the research trajectory, we sometimes used *exploratory research* to comprehend collaborative practice patterns, generate ideas about the observed facts and delve into a research problem or issue where there were few or no prior studies to which we could turn for information about the issue or problem (Collis and Hussey, 2014). Exploratory research determines whether current theories or ideas might be applied to the case under investigation and whether new theories or concepts should be established (Collis and Hussey, 2014). By finalising exploratory research, we developed new MRTs. Using descriptive analysis, we aimed to obtain information about the characteristics of an aspect of our interest—what the features were and how they came to be (Collis and Hussey, 2014). The book is also structured according to an interpretivist approach as we aimed to find meaning in our former data, observations and research (see Fulton, Kuit, Sanders and Smith, 2013). We thus explore and reflectively evaluate interprofessional practice and discover 'what' the phenomenon's characteristics are and 'how' we promote a better standard of care. Moving forward, we used *analytic or explanatory research* to learn why the fact of interest was happening by analysing the causal relations between the observed facts (Collis and Hussey, 2014).

There is a plethora of methodological approaches available, and the specific choices that we ultimately made were based on the ontological, epistemological and deontological frameworks of social research. Whatever method we adopted—whether descriptive or exploratory analysis—the individual studies helped us generate theories to explain the social world (see Clark et al., 2021). Concepts are fundamental to the generation of views, which are how we make sense of our social world, for instance, authority, social control or status (see Clark et al., 2021).

In our social research on interprofessional practice, the concepts of interprofessional collaboration, communication bottlenecks, periphery or centrality in knowledge management emerged. As further developed in this book, we extracted MRTs to explain the social aspects of interprofessional practice. A *theory* clarifies particular events or patterns observed as regularities (Clark et al., 2021). For example, *what* are the magnitudes of the regular interprofessional practice network observed in healthcare settings? The other *concepts* that were investigated throughout were (1) *professionalism,* which refers to how healthcare professionals should use their skills to create and preserve good relations with their colleagues (General Medical Council, 2022), and (2) *collaborative practice,* which offers a way to value the abilities, knowledge and contributions of our co-workers (NMC, 2015). Our *conceptions* partly derive from Maslow's need for self-actualisation through pursuing a sense of community in the teams where we worked (see McLeod, 2018). Our research aimed to *reduce social disparities, promote social inclusions and enhance team collaboration* (see Lairumbi et al., 2008).

Another critical aspect of the research was taking a self-reflective stance. This aspect was necessary since our values had some bearing on the decisions we made regarding our social studies, comprising the selection of the topic, the construction of the research question, the election of methodology and study design, and the execution of data gathering, analysis and conclusions (Clark et al., 2021). In particular, we concur that researchers must know how their value judgements influence their work (Clark et al., 2021). They should be particularly cautious about the risk that their value judgements prevent them from actively seeking and considering facts that might challenge their preconceived notions (Clark et al., 2021). Moreover, where necessary, they should be prepared to articulate and defend the evaluative stances that guide their work (Clark et al., 2021).

The choice of social network analysis (SNA) to research the topics explored by the selected studies was dictated by the need to explore the crucial and critical implications of work relationships without being swayed by the social desirability bias of responders in providing the 'expected answer' in collaborative care. Another risk is the researcher's Hawthorne bias of capturing salient and regional social phenomena that can quickly emerge because of the research and survey methods used (Jones, 1992). Instead, *indirect* research methods of social phenomena—in this instance, collaborative care in healthcare settings through sociometric analysis of interpersonal choices—can reduce social desirability bias while extracting salient points concerning social collaboration (see Tan et al., 2022).

Theoretical framework

The theoretical framework of the adopted social analysis and social networks is *relational sociology*, which uses quantitative and qualitative statistical analysis of ego networks, complemented by participant observation, ethnography and the like (Fuhse, 2015). Social networks and collaborative practice are levers in healthcare services to promote patient care and adhere to healthcare organisations' local governance of information and knowledge management. Social collaboration theories suggest that, without collaboration, specific aims cannot be fulfilled (e.g., patient care in a hospital); since other professionals have the same purpose (e.g., nurses and doctors collaborate on patient health), the aim is collective and can be fulfilled concurrently by more than one person (see Malhi and Malhi, 1999).

Harrison White, one of the precursors of relational sociology, introduced the idea that social networks are formed by people or categories of people who create more intense links with persons of the same type (professional, social, organisational and others), thus generating denser networks compared to individuals from different classes who form less concentrated ties and networks (Fuhse, 2015). This theory links to that of social systems.

This book has been informed by von Bertalanffy's (1969, 1975) *system theory*, which postulated that a system is an organised whole characterised by its components' interactions. Individuals, groups and institutions are organised in social systems in such a way as to produce an ordered web of interactions that forms a whole (Merriam-Webster Dictionary, 2022). If social systems can communicate with their surroundings and constituents, they can continue to operate (von Bertalanffy, 1969, 1972). A social system is also an assembly of individuals with specific skills that work together as a unit (Watzlawick, Bevelas and Jackson, 1967). For instance, a healthcare team comprises individuals who cooperate in treating a patient and have varied tasks (e.g., nurses, physicians, occupational therapists). Systems dynamics can be visualised in network configurations.

Moreno's (1937) sociogram theory provides an impetus for understanding teams, their interactions and their visual arrangement. Asking each team member about their connection with others is one way to examine social groupings (Moreno, 1937, 1941). The goal of group analysis is to classify the team members' positions within the groups and the functions of the groups within the community (Moreno, 1937, 1941).

Complex social systems are networks of collective behaviours with enough internal coordination and integration to make member behaviour look synchronised and orchestrated (Crossley, 2008). Social networks are patterns of interaction, guidance, communication and sustenance among the participants of the social system (Valente, 1996). SNA is used to statistically examine social networks, including communication forms and procedures, liking and disliking tendencies and the degree of interpersonal links (American Psychological Association [APA], 2022).

The trajectory used for discovery

The book forms a pathway conducive to a change in interprofessional practice. Although not individually classifiable as action research, the global intent is to highlight aspects of collaborative practice that propose a theory of evolution in transformative research. These are academic publications and instances of qualitative and mixed-method research. When a *deductive research approach* was taken, the initial step was to start from a theoretical social framework; the aim was to use what is known or emerging from research outcomes produced by the collected data to generate a hypothesis or several of them, which could confirm or reject the initial theory (Clark et al., 2021). When an inductive research approach was applied, a theory (or a set of MRTs) was extracted from the research outcomes (Clark et al., 2021). We used some stages of transformative research (TR) according to ethical guidelines to improve social justice and human rights (Mertens, 2017). TR should be culturally sensitive to the community where the research is conducted and should address the disparities within it (Mertens, 2017).

Therefore, like the network analysis of interprofessional power balance or imbalance, our book explored methods to highlight the interpersonal constraints that hinder social justice and health or, instead, the areas or needs that require improvement in this direction. Hence, similar to TR, the book considers a community's strengths or limitations to understand and address possible solutions to social disparities (Mertens, 2017). The transformational paradigm and the conceptual model underpinning it provide a framework for focussing on social discrimination and unfairness using culturally sensitive solutions and mixed methods (Mertens, 2017). Similarly to TR, the book aims to transform our understanding of an idea fundamentally, producing a paradigm shift or opening new horizons (Gravem et al., 2017).

The findings of this book are built on the knowledge we acquired from participating in interprofessional teams of HCPs in our work practice or multidisciplinary teams at university. The ultimate goal of our research was to benefit healthcare workers and their companies. Once a problem has been recognised and further studies identified why it remains a concern, the necessary solution must be discovered and implemented progressively (Nikolou-Walker and Lavery, 2009). Our research thus complies with Gibbon's concept of Mode 2 knowledge generated by addressing problems or issues in practice; as such, it draws from various disciplines and approaches (Maxwell, 2019). Mode 2 knowledge production (1) is produced in the *setting of utilisation* following the guidelines of the practice that governs a particular discipline and problem solving, which is focused around a specific purpose; (2) it is *transdisciplinary* as although the knowledge was generated in a particular setting, it develops its own unique theoretical construction, research methods and way of application, thus, through a cumulative effect it can be applied into different directions; (3) *heterogeneity* means a high number of potential settings where knowledge can be generated; (4) *social accountability and reflexivity* mean that researchers are active agents in the description and resolution of problems, but through reflexivity, they evaluate their functioning and the impact of their research which is analysed from its beginning, and (5) *quality control* means checking if the research outcome is of social interest and determining if the study will be socially suitable (Gibbons et al., 2014).

Our research was also a method for developing new knowledge, while evaluation was a systematic approach to confirming the worth of a project, strategy, action, innovation or other comparable entity to guide decision-making (Mertens, 2009). At the same time, our evaluation emphasised the importance of *assessing* as a method of systematic enquiring and using techniques that prioritised stakeholder involvement (see Mertens, 2009). Moreover, we used criteria to determine the quality, including the usefulness of the research, its practicability and ownership (e.g., results, outcomes) (see Mertens, 2009).

The axiological research paradigm suggests that principled research should advance social legitimacy and civil rights (Mertens, 2017). Understanding what it means to be culturally aware in the areas where we work; resolving inequities; acknowledging the community's strengths, abilities and resiliency; and offering justice to its people are the beginning points for ethics in research (Mertens, 2017). We were given a framework by the transformational paradigm and its philosophical tenets for addressing social injustice and unfairness in interprofessional teams (see Mertens, 2017). Because of this, several social justice and power dynamics were present in the scenarios captured in this book, including those between caregivers and patients being cared for, caregivers and researchers, patients and researchers, and interprofessional team members.

Therefore, the book can somehow be interpreted to be endorsing *some* theoretical framework of *action research*, such as (1) aiming to extract knowledge to solve a problem for the client and provide a scientific solution; (2) investigating the whole, complex problem but making it simple enough to be understood by everyone and (3) planning future changes in social systems that are suitable for organisations (Collis and Hussey, 2014).

Conclusions

The studies we selected to support the book chapters will illustrate the dynamic interplay supported by Schön's (1991) reflective practice between *reflection in action* and *reflection on action*. We conducted *reflection in action* by exploring our ongoing interprofessional experiences and research pathways, pondering on our interprofessional researchable topics, deciding how to act and using our expertise to generate robust research findings, relying on continuous work-based learning (WBL) to comprehend and investigate the social networks in interprofessional practice in the real-world in real-time (see Schön, 1991).

When each publication was completed, it became *a reflection on action*, the initial stage for further research in interprofessional practice. This prompted us to explore interprofessional teams deeply, use our former inductive and deductive analysis to collate new research evidence, generate new theoretical perspectives as MRTs and help create proposals and guidelines aimed at policymakers (see Schön, 1991; Table 1.1; Figure 1.5.).

Table 1.1. – Our reflective cycle was adjusted according to Schön's (1991) model.

Reflection stage	Content	Our applications
Reflection in action (while happening)	The actual event	Observing and participating in interprofessional teams guided WBL[a] to use research for suggesting changes.
	Considering it when it was occurring	Reflecting on the natural world as a WBL ongoing experience.
	Choosing how to respond at the moment	Improving observation, reflection and analysis methods according to interprofessional scenarios and new WBL.
	Acting without delay	The research was finalised once the methods were considered suitable to extract the desired outcomes.

Reflection stage	Content	Our applications
Reflection on action (after it happened)	Reflecting on an event that has occurred	The findings, interprofessional scenarios, reflections, research methods and outcomes from previous research were reconsidered and accrued with novel insights emerging from each research stage.
	What would I do otherwise if the situation recurred?	Providing guidelines that could appeal to policymakers, improving research methods and observations, and reinforcing research validity and transferability.
	Acquiring new knowledge and/or theoretical views that enlighten reality and facilitate the processing of actions	Outcomes generated MRTs that could be used by policymakers who want to make a change in interprofessional teams.

ªWBL = Work-Based Learning

How chapters were structured

The current book's chapters are organised in a way that presents the following stages:

1) The bibliographic reference to the selected study.
2) Our reflection in action about work-based learning during our daily practice that triggered our interest in researching a specific area.
3) The theoretical background that led to the research with citations of seminal authors and publications from other authors.
4) The outcomes of the study.
5) The MRTs extractable from the chapter were corroborated and developed from our previous research and published articles, books and book chapters.
6) Our reflection on action on how we applied the findings in the chapters and how they guided our practice with hints on policies and corporate governance (Figure 1.5).

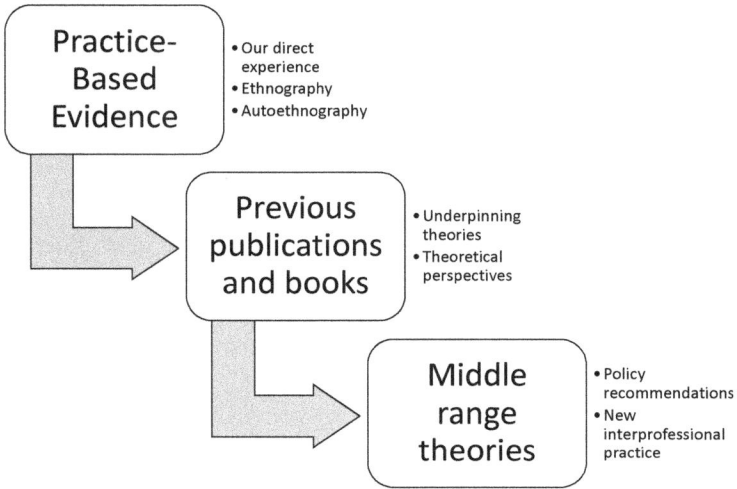

Figure 1.5. – A process of how the models and middle-range theories developed in the current book.

The aim of future actions, bringing a team together, does not always depend on how much the system collaborates with us to assess the outcome; there will always be grey areas we need to explain in our professional challenge. The timeline can stretch beyond our desire to bring about an immediate result as there are different methods to approach the topic, given the context. We are presenting an account of what might serve our purpose best (Figure 1.6).

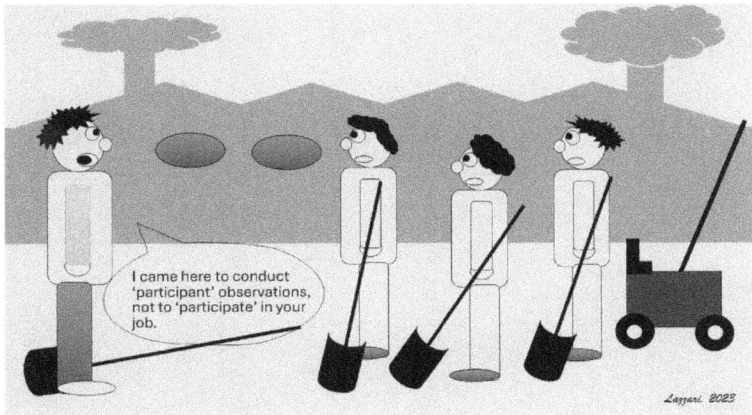

Figure 1.6. – Participant ethnographic observation entails participating in all or most activities of the observed group to extract its salient characteristics.

CHAPTER 2

Interprofessional Teams

Abstract

The current chapter is based on the critical evaluation of the publication Lazzari, C. (2019) 'Interprofessional education and practice and the application of social network analysis' *Cientperiodique Medicine*, 5(4), pp. 1–12. This study explores the characteristics of functional and dysfunctional interprofessional teams. We will investigate the main bottlenecks in interprofessional practice.

Reflections *in* action

The following paragraph is an excerpt from our diary, which we kept while conducting this public study and working in interprofessional teams. The following extract encapsulates the issue that prompted our research question and the writing of the paper. It captures, ad verbatim, our conversation with our supervisors or colleagues.

> «Working in multidisciplinary teams as participants, we feel that our information exchanges through communication influence each other and the dynamics of our team. It is an all-encompassing experience. The information we receive and give in our teams is essential for the function of the group and the understanding and care of our customers. However, we perceive that sometimes, this balance is skewed, and there are bottlenecks in information exchange.

Some information does not circulate among all team members. Instead, we believe our knowledge exchanges should be balanced and not favour some while keeping others out of the loop. If someone does not integrate into the team, this process has consequences on our global actions as an interprofessional team. A peripheral person in the group probably has the most important information we need to work on, but that individual is not encouraged to share it. At other times, the team seems too reliant on being guided by the most high-ranking persons and does not empower itself to be more proactive in decision-making. We shall all be accountable for our actions and do our part in interprofessional teams. Each of us can make a change» (Table 2.1).

Table 2.1. – Reflection in action in teamwork strategies.

The actual event	Considering it when it was occurring	Settings where applied	Acting without delay (motto)	Choosing how to respond at the moment
Bottlenecks in healthcare information.	The information does not circulate among all team members.	Morning handovers and multidis-ciplinary team meetings (MDT) for patients' discussions.	Act and speak now.	We encourage all team members to share their opinions and observations during MDT meetings.
Peripheral hubs of persons who do not partake in multidis-ciplinary decisions.	Not all profes-sionals involved in patient care share their knowledge for teams' decisions.	Electronic patient records (EPR) are the best platform to reduce isolated hubs of professionals.	Make yourself known; say what you know now.	Each morning at handovers, team members read recent electronic patient records (EPR); every team member is essential to reach a working approach to the case.

The actual event	Considering it when it was occurring	Settings where applied	Acting without delay (motto)	Choosing how to respond at the moment
Power skewness by solely relying on the high-ranking team members.	Seniority and expertise are the responsibility of amalgamating team members.	Day-by-day team decisions.	No one is 'more' important.	Shared leadership means anyone is actively accountable for a patient's care without delegating duties and responsibilities to others.

Study justification

Since we participated in interprofessional teams and progressively developed interprofessional theories in healthcare settings, we could identify more intensely the similarities between care teams and any social and living systems. Our observations in professional settings compelled us to read more about the systems theory we approached years after graduating. In the 1980s, we began reading and learning about systemic approaches. In 1986, one of us published the first paper on social systems and organisational conflicts, which was presented at the International Meeting of Cybernetics and Systems in Namur, Belgium, entitled *Power and Conflicts in Complex Systems and the Ethics of Human Relations Explained by Cybersystemic Models* (Lazzari, 1986). When we embarked on interprofessional research, there was limited literature on using the concepts explored in the current chapter and its underpinning theory. Thinking of interprofessional teams as social networks and using social network analysis and ethnographic research to extract their dynamics were new avenues for studying this topic (Lazzari, 2019b).

We have recognised the value of diverse teams' feedback-giving-and-receiving processes. According to social systems theory, society is a dynamic and linked network that includes people and their perspectives about the entity (such as a country, organisation, setting, and so on) that unites them and their interactions to sustain their joint venture (Gibson, 2022). Typically, the 19th century is where the method's roots may be located, especially in the writings of French social scientist

Émile Durkheim and English philosopher and sociologist Herbert Spencer (Gibson, 2022).

Because of our studies in medicine or our healthcare or academic background, we could recognise how the concept of interacting cells in human organs relates to the idea of networking living beings in human societies. According to the biologist von Bertallanfy (1969), the trait shared by all living organisms (biological organs, social groups, and so on) is their organisation. This concept means that the modes of operation of higher-level societies cannot be explained by the aggregate of their components' characteristics and configurations of action when those components are considered in isolation but rather by the relations between them. People interact with one another and share information within their social systems; these last are defined and shaped by these interactions (von Bertalanffy, 1972). The mathematician Weiner (1954), the founder of cybernetics, introduced the concept of feedback: fundamental to all organisms, either living societies or machines, feedback is the communication sent and received back (feedback) between units of the organism, the community and the device. To remain functional, social systems' members should be able to give and receive information and feedback from other members of that and other systems (von Bertalanffy, 1972; Weiner, 1954, 2013, 2019). How are these concepts related to interprofessional practice?

According to the 2022 edition of the *Cambridge Dictionary Online*, a system is a group of related items or humans that act together and have a specific purpose. According to the *Encyclopedia Britannica* (Gibson, 2019), social systems theory studies society as the composition of individuals and their beliefs and how they interact, for example, as a country. A characteristic of social systems is their power to adapt to the environment (e.g., social, political, and biological) by changing their level of integration (Gibson, 2019).

Once we collected our data and observations, we merged them into a unitary model to attract possible healthcare policymakers and highlight areas of reinforcement in interprofessional practice to advance healthcare's condition and configuration. To offer an overarching model from our research, we crafted several middle-range theories (MRTs) of interprofessional practices extracted from exploring a specific phenomenon or experience from research, literature or practice (Roy, 2014). MRTs synthesise concepts into knowledge that can be generalised beyond a given situation and serve as seeds of further knowledge development, including designing and testing interventions in healthcare practice (Roy, 2014). An MRT begins with observable phenomena and abstracts from them to provide general claims that data can validate (Merton, 1968).

The theories or reflections highlighted in the current and subsequent chapters and publications also comply with WBL and experiences. WBL entails altering the conventional views and perspectives of the workplace and working knowledge (Nikolou-Walker and Garnett, 2004). As a result, engaging in reflective practice helped us better understand our role in our workplace while raising issues about our identity and the extent to which we needed personal growth (Nikolou-Walker and Garnett, 2004). During the research leading to the compilation of the book, we proposed a set of MRTs of interprofessional practice to provide a new interprofessional model and extend our insights into social phenomena in healthcare organisations. The current chapter is based on extracting the MRTs of what is noticeable in interprofessional teams regarding their interpersonal interactions and information exchange.

Background

The current chapter summarises the salient theories that subsequently formed the basis of our study of interprofessional practice. Several concepts are elaborated on throughout this chapter and further developed in the following ones. This chapter summarises what several authors have identified as the characteristics of interprofessional practice. For instance, several sources cite that an interprofessional approach enhances satisfaction with teamwork, which may result in better quality patient care (GMC, 2017). Another advantage of training healthcare professionals in collaborative practice is that they become mindful of their and their colleagues' actions during reciprocal interactions, reinforce information exchange and grow more connected with the needs of their shared clients (WHO, 2010).

Conversely, conflicts within teams in healthcare organisations can reduce effective patient care and harm treatment quality (Lazzari, 2004). In addition, the findings derived from our research are based on practice. We wanted to extract conclusions that could have an academic impact (Costley and Fulton, 2018; Costley, Elliott and Gibbs, 2010) while attracting the relevant parties and policymakers in the healthcare area.

A concept frequently used in the book and constantly explored in other publications on the same topic is 'social network'—a group of individuals and the relationships they share (Wasserman and Faust, 1994). Social networks can be studied using targeted research strategies and ethnographic observation (Lazzari, 2019). Social Network Analysis (SNA), for example, is a method in which team dynamics are qualitatively and quantitatively described using pictorial representations of them (qualitative analysis) or by capturing and measuring the intensity of the interpersonal bonds between the people comprising a network, either their number or their strength (quantitative analysis) (Scott, 2017; Figure 2.1.).

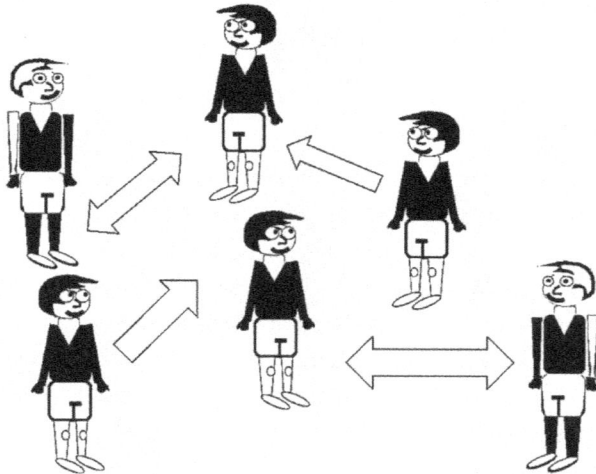

Figure 2.1. – Schematic representation of a social network.

One of the research strategies that helped us understand teams and their dynamics was immersing ourselves in the *culture* we wanted to understand—a process called ethnography or anthropology (see Lazzari, 2019). The *Merriam-Webster Dictionary* (2022) identifies culture as a group of collective views, principles, goals and customs that define an organisation's structure. Teams in clinical settings represent the culture of public or private hospitals. Because clinical practitioners have various duties and diverse expectations, improved social research can be conducted by understanding their communal experiences (Passini, 2010) and cultures.

Margaret Mead (2004), a notable anthropological researcher, believed that personal experience is never adequate to develop an appropriate worldview; to build a proper worldview, according to her, one must understand other people's perspectives; humans, she believed, can learn from each other. By creating social systems, individuals from disparate backgrounds can combine their abilities to benefit humankind (Mead, 2004).

Therefore, another step in investigating teamwork and team dynamics was to study groups as systems. Von Bertalanffy's (1969) General System Theory states that living organisms are systems of units linked by mutual exchanges and communication; they remain alive and functional if they can share information with their environment and between their separate sections (e.g., cells, organs, groups, species). We believe that interprofessional teams of the HCP system can achieve their clinical goals through constant communication with their members. According to von Bertalanffy (1969), a system is an organised whole composed of interacting components. It can also be defined as a group of persons with specific characteristics categorised by the relationships that each element or member of the system has with others (Watzlawick, Bevelas and Jackson, 1967).

A team of HCPs comprises persons with specific areas of expertise (e.g., nurses, doctors, occupational therapists, clinical psychologists) who interact by exchanging information and knowledge between and among them, as well as with the hospital, the customers, the patient's families and the community teams. The characteristics of social systems include their interconnection, as a change in one section of a system affects the whole organisation (Watzlawick, Bevelas and Jackson, 1967). This characteristic of *unity* or *wholeness* can be manifested in varying degrees (Watzlawick, Bevelas and Jackson, 1967). For example, our interprofessional teams sometimes had moments of impasse when some vital information about a patient's care or learner's progress was not circulated among all the team affiliates. All associates of open social systems are also linked and regulated by *feedback* mechanisms, meaning that they influence and are influenced by one another (Watzlawick, Bevelas and Jackson, 1967).

Interprofessional practice and communication in HCPs are represented by specific configurations of their social networks (Shoham et al., 2016). In communal language, a piece of information refers to the facts (e.g., clinical data about a patient, student records) or opinions (e.g., a professional's diagnosis of a case, marks on school assignments) that are given or received during our life; information can be derived from others or any form of media (e.g., television, radio, smartphones, electronic data and so on) (Slamecka, 2022). We thus felt that *any characteristic or deviation from the normal flow of communication and interaction exchanges in interprofessional teams is translated into specific network configurations; these arrangements can be observed and measured* (Lazzari, 2019).

Methodology of the public works

A better understanding of teams, interactions and pictorial configu-rations began with Moreno's (1937, 1941) sociograms. Moreno suggests two effective methods for studying social groups: (1) asking each team member to answer questions about their relationships with others and (2) using the observational method, which involves studying the group relationships from outside (Moreno, 1937, 1941). We utilised both methods throughout our research on interprofessional practice, asking team members whom they selected to request or provide information on patient care (Lazzari and Rabottini, 2021). We were also participant observers of these or similar teams when, for ethical reasons, we had to separate ourselves from our research's target population (Lazzari, 2019). We focused on observable interactions and behaviours because, as Moreno (1937, 1941) suggests, team members might not always disclose their feelings about one another. The analysis of groups aims to categorise the position of team members and the role of the groups in society (Moreno, 1937, 1941).

The constituents (in our case, HCPs) of social networks are referred to as nodes or actors, and they may take the form of individuals or organisations; the connections, or ties, that exist between the nodes are responsible for the flow of information and actions and are capable of taking a variety of forms (Yang, Keller and Zheng, 2016). When data are shared, resources or knowledge are exchanged, or the subjects in the network complete cooperative actions, the communications and relationships between units or persons in a social network are typically depicted by double-headed arrows—this is a give-and-take feedback process between sender and receiver of the communication (Yang, Keller and Zheng, 2016). However, when the interaction is unilateral, a single-headed arrow connects the two parties—in this case, the sender is deprived of the feedback process about its communicated data or shared action (Yang, Keller and Zheng, 2016; Figure 2.2.).

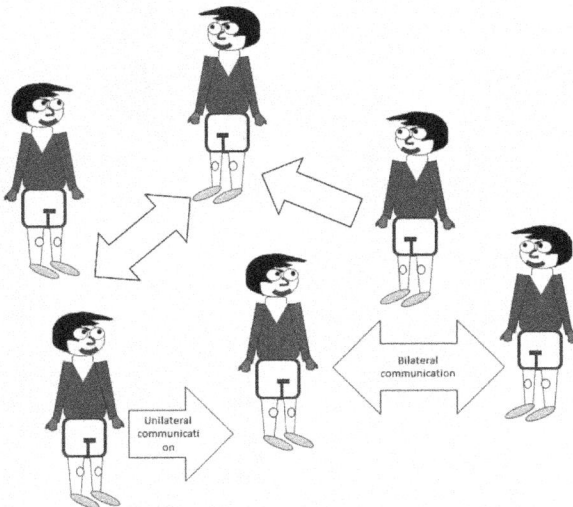

Figure 2.2. – Unilateral (single-headed arrow) or a bilateral (double-headed arrow) interchange of communication and information in social networks.

Suppose a team member has the highest number of incoming and outgoing links with others compared with the rest of the team. In that case, that person is considered a gatekeeper and holds (or occupies) a central position in the network as it is equally a sender and receiver in the communication process (Lazzari, 2018b). Therefore, to capture which HCP plays a crucial role in interprofessional teams, the parameter most used is the *degree of centrality* (Prell, 2012). Many incoming connections (knowledge, resources, data and other assets) acquired by one individual from other team members identify that person's *prestige level, denominated in-degree centrality* subcategory (Prell, 2012). On the other hand, the subcategory called *out-degree centrality* suggests many connections between persons, also signifying the *expansiveness* of those persons with outgoing links (Prell, 2012). An interprofessional social network of HCPs is composed of persons who have unilateral (represented by a single-headed arrow in a social network graph) and/ or bilateral (double-headed arrow) interchanges of communication and information (see Prell, 2012; Figure 2.3).

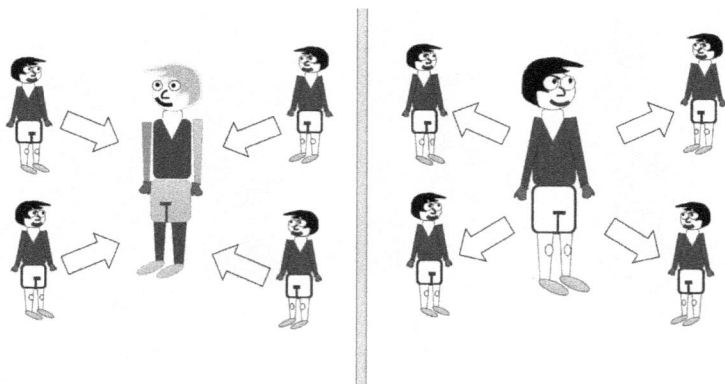

Figure 2.3. – In in-degree centrality (left), a team member receives more information from others or does so more frequently; s/he is a high receiver. In out-degree centrality (right), a team member provides more information to others or does so more regularly; s/ he is a high sender.

Findings

In the research presented in the current chapter, we identified five significant configurations of interprofessional networks from our ethnographic observations of healthcare teams and their impact on teamwork (Lazzari, 2019):

a) In the *isolation-type network,* although some HCPs possess critical information for the team and patient care, they seldom participate in team choices and discussions; the team does not appear to encourage these healthcare providers to share their information with the group, resulting in a knowledge management gaps in patient care; collegial participation is crucial during multidisciplinary (MDT) meetings where each team member can share what s/he knows about communal patients to promote their safety and care policies; if some member (including the most high-ranking) is isolated in the network, the outcome is missed patient care and information, and lost data about patient progress and current presentation;

b) In the *decentralised-type network,* some professionals share essential information exclusively with close affiliates or acquaintances, excluding other team members (for example, more junior HCPs); in this case, as well, there are gaps in information flow; the risk is that vital information and handovers are not circulated within a team, jeopardising patient health and safety;

c) The *hyper-centralised network* is where all information and knowledge management are the prerogatives or originate from a few professionals in central or high-ranking positions, primarily gatekeepers (e.g., senior nurse, senior doctor, senior psychologist); there is a high intensity of the outdegree centrality of information; however, this condition might decrease the likelihood that other professionals could equally contribute to the whole team's activity and decisions with their share of information; therefore, patients cannot receive integrated care, and vital advice about proper management; primary data are lost as some HCPs cannot communicate and are not invited by centralised professionals;

d) The *overloading network* occurs when one person has a high intensity of inbound communication and advice (e.g., their team might consider them the least qualified in the group, they do not cover more high-ranking positions, or they are the information or decision gatekeepers). This person usually receives information, advice, resources and duties from any team member, but s/he cannot reciprocate in kind; this network shows a high in-degree centrality; the risk is that the team might not receive guidance from this person or facilitate feedback from him/her to ensure that the information, advice or duty the team provided and assigned was valid, understood, applied or undertaken; when high-ranking and more experienced HCPs are overloaded with unidirectional communication (policies, emails, urgent requests), they cannot redistribute duties as message senders might not ensure that feedback communication occurs;

e) *The clustering network* occurs when professionals with similar educational backgrounds or knowhow levels tend to interact more tightly than other HCPs in the team; the risk is that those estranged by the central hubs might not usually have an impact on knowledge-sharing and decision-making in their interprofessional team, although they might be equally crucial for customer care; when occurring in hospitals, separated groups creating hubs allocated to the same customer might be unable to integrate care and information thus missing data for patient assessment and interventions.

Conclusions and middle-range theories

It is argued that applying academic skills to 'real-world' situations brings theory out of the classroom and onto people's desks at work or other places where they want to learn and apply knowledge (Nikolou-Walker, 2007). To generate MRTs, we linked our published research to the findings of the current chapter to trace our professional and research development.

MRT-1

Interprofessional teams are more than the mere aggregate of their specific members. Instead, they can exist for their goals as long as interchanges among all interprofessional team members occur according to three significant aspects: (1) *equifinality*, whose aim is for all team members to participate in a common goal, (2) *impartiality*, in the sense that each team member is indispensable for the achievement of a common goal, and (3) *equipotential bonding*, which indicates that each team fellow is a carrier of critical information for joint customer assessment and care planning. The flow of information should thus not have any peaks that focus only on a few team members, while the team ensures that knowledge and information are circulated and reviewed constantly; in functional teams, there is a balance between information senders and receivers (Lazzari, 2008; Lazzari and Masiello, 2016; Lazzari, 2019). We also observed that team participation might continue beyond face-to-face encounters as each team member might tend to mentally elaborate interprofessional interactions into an infinite number of possibilities of the kind 'if I do this, then they...'. This is a form of social mindfulness where interactive (if-then) scenarios are mentally rehearsed to establish teamwork's best course of action. We might also hypothesise that interprofessional exchanges require this mental preparation to allow each team member to predict others' reactions to their past, present or future actions (Figure 2.4.).

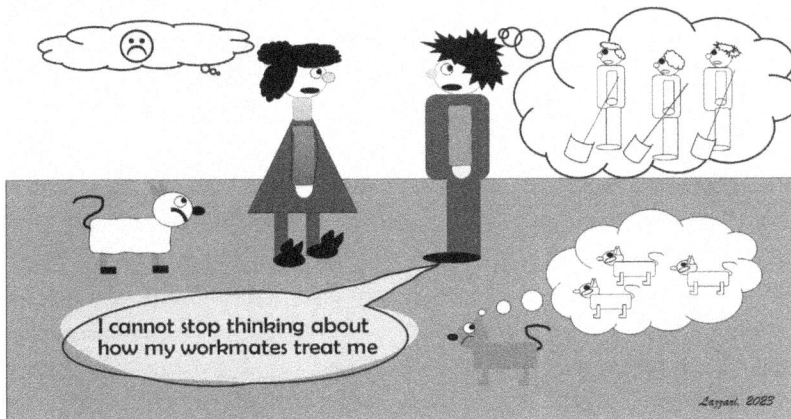

Figure 2.4. – Each team member might continue pondering about interprofessional interactions and rehearse possible mental scenarios of how others might react to their actions and words when face-to-face.

MRT-2

Interprofessional teams with an intense centralisation of information flow that excludes the peripheral HCPs might risk not having everyone on the same page regarding vital customer information (Lazzari, McAleer, Nusair and Rabottini, 2022). There will be bottlenecks in collaborative care; such a team might quickly tip into chaos and impact the quality of interactions with patients by increasing the likelihood of professional malpractice or interpersonal conflicts (Lazzari, 2006; Lazzari and Masino, 2006).

When social systems grow more chaotic, they show increased entropy, which measures a (social) system's capacity to forecast the possible states of its internal configuration (Wiener, 1954). Entropy is deemed low if the future state or any potential upcoming scenario is largely foreseeable and vice versa; consequently, a system with low entropy is considered structured and, by inference, more desirable and predictable (Wiener, 1954). Weiner (1954), the founder of cybernetics, also postulates that when entropy increases, social systems naturally tend to move from a state of organisation to a condition of chaos and repetitiveness. The outcome in interprofessional teams with high entropy negatively impacts customers' health (Lazzari and Masino, 2015) and generates less than optimal communication in helping relationships (Lazzari, 2008).

MRT-3

To restore order and ensure intense interprofessional communication, training HCPs to communicate in interprofessional teams is paramount (Lazzari, McAleer and Rabottini, 2021). Training equips workers with the necessary abilities to complete their obligations and tasks (Nikolou-Walker and Meaklim, 2007). An activity that removes skill and knowledge gaps might be claimed to solve a performance issue when these shortcomings lead to errors, flaws, excesses and so on (Nikolou-Walker and Meaklim, 2007). Hence, the assessment of interprofessional behaviour through ethnographic observations will guide policymakers and clinical governance in the process of unobtrusive reviews and audits of procedures meant to enhance the safety of patients and treatment quality (Lazzari, 2018b).

Our reflection *on* action, professional growth and a way to change

When we finished this research phase, we believed we could better configure interprofessional practice and have more theoretical and practical knowledge. By developing the findings into theoretical and systemic statements, we thought we could now approach policymakers to explore the points of interprofessional improvement, reduce gaps in information sharing and, thus, enhance customer care. We also noticed that interprofessional teams rely on information gatekeepers who direct most of the information flow and knowledge management. These individuals tend to be the most high-ranking or experienced figures. However, it is essential to include other professionals in the information and knowledge management networks when they occupy peripheral areas of interprofessional networks; this adjustment will restore a vital balance between information senders and receivers. As information gatekeepers, we constantly endeavour to communicate with all our team members. Each member of our teams can and is encouraged to offer valuable knowledge and information to the troupe. We regularly promote those at the network's periphery or those less involved in the team to share their experiences and communicate with the rest of the group. Missing the chain of interprofessional exchanges can severely affect the comprehensiveness of care, patient safety, or student progress at school.

The next stage of the research

This chapter explored the theoretical and applicative aspects of the network analysis of interprofessional teams. At this stage, the research was applied in the targeted fields and settings using more robust methodological instruments to capture and measure the network of work distribution in interprofessional teams. Once the theoretical understanding of the topic was completed, the next stage was to apply the findings in teams and understand how the distribution of tasks and expertise within interprofessional teams impacted the type and amount of care offered to hospital inpatients. The setting was dementia wards, where persons with multiple needs require integrated care from their caregivers.

CHAPTER 3

Teamwork and Patients

Abstract

The current chapter has been created by exploring the findings of the publication Lazzari, C., Kotera, Y. and Thomas, H. (2019) 'Social network analysis of dementia wards in psychiatric hospitals to explore the advancement of personhood in patients with Alzheimer's disease', *Current Alzheimer Research*, 16(6), pp. 505–517. The project aimed to explore labour distribution in multidisciplinary teams, the patient's role in interprofessional teams, and how multitasking team members might benefit the whole organisation.

Our reflection *in* action

The following paragraph is a quote from our chronicle, which we kept when conducting this public study and working in interprofessional teams. This excerpt details the issue that prompted our research question and the writing of the chapter. It is an ad verbatim extraction of our conversation with our colleagues in dementia wards.

> «Some of us are working in a dementia ward. We see that any team member actively provides holistic care to patients with Alzheimer's. Some nurses go the extra mile and attend to patients' physical, personal and social needs. These wards usually scored highly during CQC (Care Quality Commission) inspections. However, we also

worked in other hospital wards (private and public) or teams. Some team members did not seem to go beyond what was strictly requested from their job description. Also, when quality time could be spent with patients or service users, some staff members preferred staying in their office or delegating what they could have quickly done to communal customers. In this case, patients did not feel motivated to engage with any staff members and spent most of their time in their rooms. When the team was not involved in face-to-face encounters with patients, these last also moved to a progressive demotivation, and the signs of institutionalisation appeared more evident» (Table 3.1).

Table 3.1. – Reflection in action in teamwork and strategies.

The actual event	Considering it when it was occurring	Settings where applied	Acting without delay (motto)	Choosing how to respond at the moment
Some team members could do more but remain unitasking.	Some team members disengage from teamwork and delegate to others.	Daily routines at the bedside and direct interactions with patients.	Help others, and don't delegate.	Team leaders should redistribute tasks and duties to engage those who want to do less.
Reduced quality of time with patients.	Some team members might assume a passive role when engaging with patients.	Ibid.	Speak with patients and engage them as equals.	Team leaders should ensure that each team member has quality time with patients and avoids idle time in the wards.

Background

Our WBL, intended to develop practical solutions in interprofessional team practice and patient care, inspired this chapter. This book borrows an essential idea from action research, where a researcher aims to learn through critical analysis of a phenomenon and to actively work towards improving practice (Nikolou-Walker and Lavery, 2009). Integrated care pathways specify, for a specific clinical condition, the duties that must be performed, the timing and order in which these obligations must be carried out, and the level of organisation required to accomplish them (Campbell et al., 1998). Integrated care may also be defined as care that is planned with individuals who work together to get to know the service users and their service providers, as well as to organise and provide assets to get the best possible results by joining their professional efforts towards a common goal (NHS Health Education England, 2022).

Visualising this cooperation is the initial stage in identifying mutuality and its blockages; consequently, social network analysis enables the construction of social maps and the extraction of centrality indicators, both of which reveal blockages in the flow of information and suggest ways to improve the efficiency of teams (Grippa et al., 2018). Integrated care in an interprofessional team refers to the coordinated actions of multiple HCPs who act either in real-time (all at the same time) or intermittently (each one at a specific and separate time or location) on a communal patient to deliver a care strategy that has been approved by the whole team (Lazzari, Kotera, Thomas and Rabottini, 2019). The interdisciplinary teams that work in Alzheimer's wards were the subject of this chapter. In these conditions, partnership and integrated teamwork are essential to address the composite demands of older persons and ensure patient-centred care (Lazzari, 2018a).

Theoretical background

This chapter's research question was: How can one understand interprofessional practice in integrated care? Goffman described healthcare organisations as 'total institutions,' suggesting that the interests of the organisation and the individual member merge in voluntary cooperation and by sharing organisational guidelines to achieve values in wellbeing and interpersonal collaboration (Goffman, 1961). Goffman (1961) became deeply interested in psychiatric hospitals from within as an observer, setting time to capture the official and unofficial behaviours of persons in these locations. The method Goffman introduced was called 'unsystematic observation' (Goffman, 1963a, 1963b; Manning, 1992). Observations of naturalistic interactions between Goffman and people were not systematic because he collected observations from as many diverse situations as possible (Goffman 1963a, 1963b; Manning, 1992). These observations were also selective, as Goffman chose to focus on detailed aspects of social interactions and ignore others; he watched people in healthcare organisations as he and they went about their normal activities, and from this viewpoint, he constructed general theories of social interactions in total institutions (e.g., hospitals, wards) (Goffman, 1969; Manning, 1992). As Goffman adds, there might be overlapping definitions of situations in which interpersonal interactions will (re)define the rules of their social engagement (Goffman, 1963a, 1963b). For instance, internal regulations in different clinical settings might establish diverse priorities that might not apply to other teams in the same or other locations.

This chapter also examined the idea of personhood, which contends that an individual with any illness has needs that must be recognised in their fullness and that are biological, psychological, social, historical, moral, theological, legal, financial and civic (Kitwood, 1997). According to Kitwood (1997), personhood is the significance or value placed on an individual by others within the framework of a relationship or link. To differentiate a specific kind of dementia support from conventional health and behavioural therapies, Tom Kitwood coined the term 'personhood' in 1988 to represent a carer focusing on communication and connection with her service user (cited in Fazio et al., 2018). For example, dementia caregivers attend to the personhood of persons with Alzheimer's (PWAs), which consists of three binding domains: biological, individual and sociologic personhood, while addressing the numerous demands of PWAs (Buron, 2008).

Similarly, the concept of person-centred care comes from Carl Rogers, who emphasises the centrality of the unique human occurrence as the cornerstone for care and its achievement as a measure of successful therapeutic acts (Fazio et al., 2018). Patients with any illnesses have a series of vital needs that can be medical (e.g., need for treatment of an underlying respiratory problem), psychological (need for emotional support for dealing with bereavement), social (e.g., need for help to access community services), religious (e.g., need for assistance to attend worship activities in the local church), legal (e.g., need for legal advice about mortgages) and financial (e.g., need for support for basic living expenses) (Hughes, 2014). Whoever attends to hospital patients or community service users and helps them with their needs must coordinate with other HCPs to provide integrated care and unitary service (Lazzari, Kotera and Thomas, 2019). In this way, personhood is reinforced by patient-centred care (Lazzari, 2018).

Local governance standards reiterate these ideals in all therapeutic settings. In the UK, CQC (Care Quality Commission) requirements and assessments apply to all care homes, services provided in patients' households, surgeries, dentists, GP (general practitioner or family doctor) services, hospitals, social services, healthcare services and other health providers (CQC, 2022). The service quality is usually rated on a scale of 'excellent' to 'inadequate' (CQC, 2022). A service that does not meet the CQC criteria risks being investigated. These are the requirements: excellence is the first value that every organisation should uphold, followed by compassion and treating everyone with respect—both patients and staff, integrity—doing the right thing, and teamwork—learning from one another to become the best one can be (CQC, 2022; Figure 3.1.).

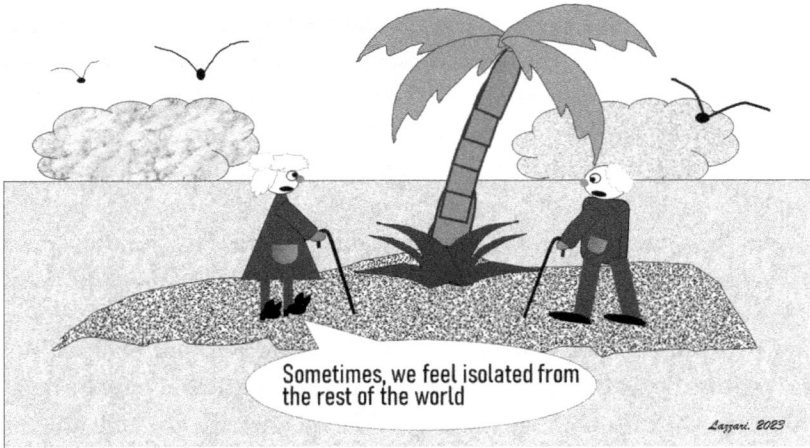

Figure 3.1. – Interprofessional teams can help frail people overcome feelings of solitude and abandonment.

Methodology

Understanding the complex networks of teams that operate in healthcare systems from an insider perspective is a milestone for knowledge and change. Ethnography offers one method for moving in this direction (Lazzari, 2018)[1]. Ethnographic research aims to better extrapolate from a culture the social data that the individuals who are part of that culture might not be aware of (Polit and Beck, 2022), such as the formation of centralised subgroups and the exclusion of other peripheral team members (Lazzari, 2019).

It has been reported that the credibility of research findings extracted from ethnographic observations can improve when the researcher spends extended periods in the setting of interest for data collection (Saldaña, 2011). Ethnography may be defined as the descriptive study of a specific human civilisation, or it can refer to the process of conducting such

---

1 Ethnography is the description of and research about societies or civilisations based on the researcher's direct experience (as in field research) and (ideally) involvement. (Reference: Americal Psychological Association (2023) *Definition of 'ethnography'*, Available at: https://dictionary.apa.org/ethnography [Accessed: 21 Aug 2023]).

research (Encyclopaedia Britannica, 2022). Contemporary ethnography almost exclusively depends on observations, necessitating the anthropologist's (or any other researcher's) thorough immersion in the culture and daily lives of their investigation's foci (Encyclopaedia Britannica, 2022).

Another method adopted was Social Network Analysis or SNA. The words 'social networks' and 'social systems' were used interchangeably to describe a set of persons linked by interactions. However, SNA can also study structures of influence, communication and perceptions of persons connected by relationships (Nimmon and Cristancho, 2019). Social network maps as sociograms visually capture connections, disconnections and the positions of influence of people within a team, with the lines of a network representing their relational ties (Nimmon, Artino and Varpio, 2019). Social network theory, which was created by the field of relational sociology, examines how a network of people's relationships are structured through various social constructs and places a focus on culture, meaning and communication; it provides insights into how the logical dynamics of teamwork relate to these social constructs (Nimmon, Artino and Varpio, 2019).

Social networks are maintained through shared communication; the analysis of these networks asks each member who are the other persons in the network with whom they have some regular interaction (Fuhse, 2015). We adapted the configuration of social networks of interprofessional practice to link persons to their clinical actions. These *two-mode social networks* can also link persons to their shared activities in their team and illustrate the division of labour, gaps in team performance or coordinated steps towards common goals (Crossley et al., 2015). SNA can be a powerful educational tool in healthcare organisations, providing a snapshot of the configuration of power dynamics and the distribution of labour in collaborative practice (Nimmon, Artino and Varpio, 2019) (Figures 3.2. and 3.3.).

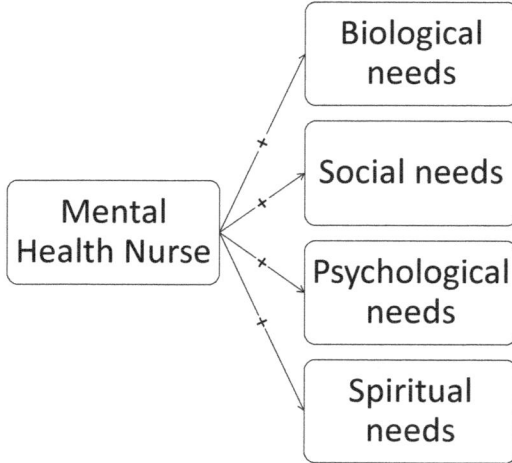

Figure 3.2. – A multitasking nurse attending to multiple patient needs.

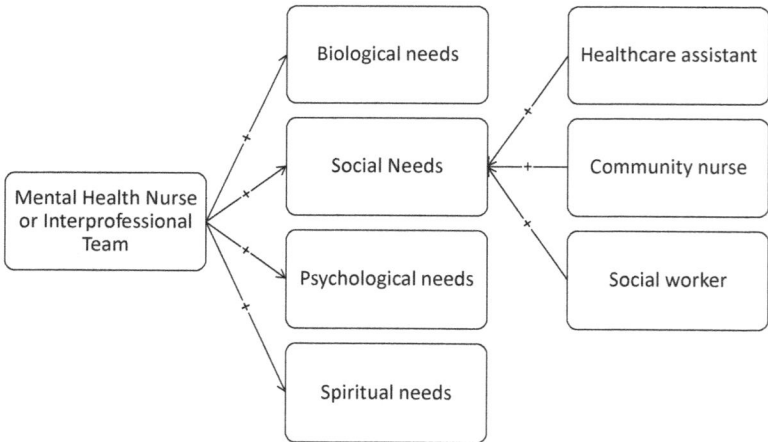

Figure 3.3. – Multitasking workers or interprofessional teams (left), unlike uni-tasking workers (right), can attend to patients' multiple needs with minimal collateral support.

Findings

When the HCPs attended to patients' *physical needs*, they provided regular physical check-ups (e.g., assessing blood pressure, blood sugar level, blood oxygen level and temperature). The other physical needs included manual handling and patient mobilisation if needed. The nurses also ensured patients' regular food and fluid intake and, with other healthcare professionals, monitored patients' bowel movements, urinary infections, signs of intoxication from accidental ingestion of any substance and side effects from medications. In dementia wards, the nurses also reduced the risk of choking and falls in patients with Alzheimer's or helped them with mobility (Figure 3.4.).

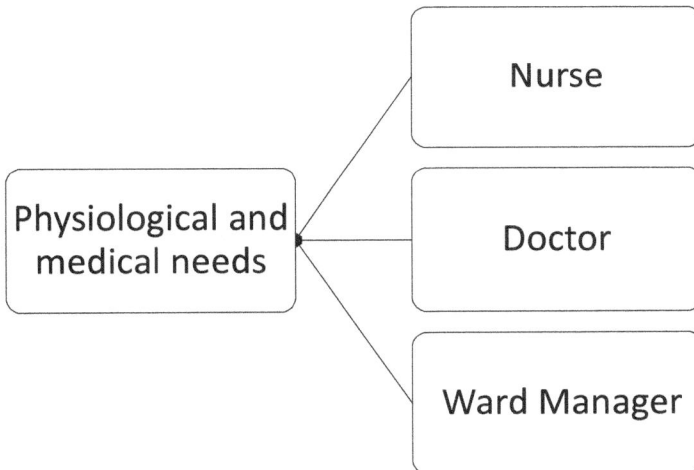

Figure 3.4. – Not all professionals are involved in addressing the physiological needs of patients.

When attending to *personal needs*, the HCPs helped patients recollect pleasant historical and personal memories and checked whether they had any spiritual needs or were church attendees to help them join them. The HCPs created dementia-friendly wards by displaying patients' photos and belongings in their rooms. They never failed to convey empathy with the patients, even after these last lost their ability to communicate and speak for themselves. When patients were silent due to dementia or did not want to verbalise their anguish, the HCPs used empathetic touch and continually engaged patients' attention. In addition, HCPs made sure that the communal areas were roomy and well-lit and that the patients had access to a large variety of items to keep themselves occupied, including an assortment of events and inspiring items (music, picture books and so on), as well as other leisure activities, such as sitting by the pool or gardening and so on (Figure 3.5.).

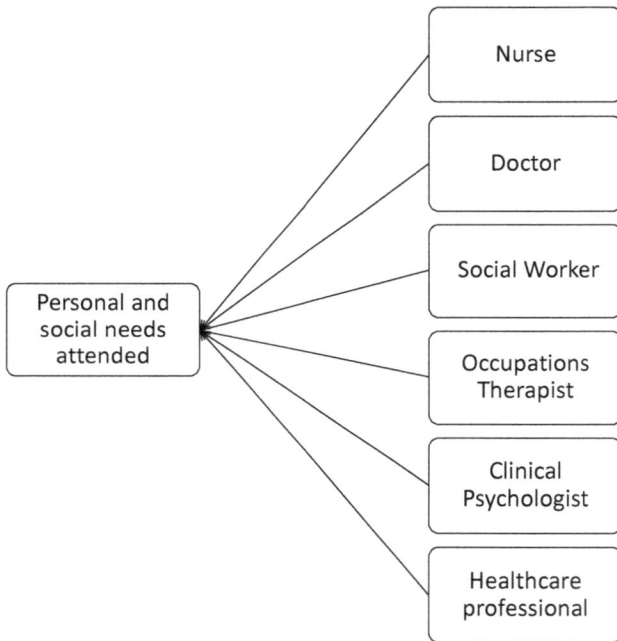

Figure 3.5. – Most HCPs could attend to the personal and social needs of patients.

When attending to patient's *social needs*, the HCPs encouraged family members to visit their hospitalised relative regularly. HCPs helped transport patients or families to and from the hospital. HCPs kept regular contact with family members via phone, informing them of the progress of their relatives. HCPs organised leave to local towns, areas and cafeterias when possible and during hospital leave. Social needs were also promoted by sensitising the local community to the desires and conditions of the patients. The patients' families were also involved in decisions concerning their care and any other aspect of the care plan, such as authorising or not resuscitation if a patient needed it.

Conclusions and pedagogical applications

SNA highlighted the social distribution of care to individual patients, captured the network of actions addressed to patients' needs and indicated routes to reinforce collaborative care (Lazzari, McAleer and Rabottini, 2022). The pedagogical approach of visualising the provision of help in healthcare networks can flag how the distribution of labour might help or hinder patients' efforts to reintegrate the distinct aspects of the self (physical, social, spiritual and individual) into a unitary whole (Lazzari, Kotera and Thomas, 2019). Moreover, SNA revealed how interprofessional teams care for different aspects of personhood and where gaps might cause fragmented care (Lazzari, Kotera and Thomas, 2019). Therefore, one may infer that all the HCPs protected the humanity of people with health issues (Lazzari, Kotera and Thomas, 2019). We supposed that the psychiatric dementia wards audited followed Kitwood's type B organisational standard, in which staff members shared their values and expertise with the rest of the team; such an environment is thought to foster joint participation in patient care when there is trust among team members, and they have had a chance to learn about the ward's routines, patients, co-workers and policies (Kitwood, 1997).

Middle-range theories

The following MRTs generated by merging the chapter's findings with our previously published research might help policymakers find the ground for addressing improvements in interprofessional practice.

MRT 1
Learning integrated care in interprofessional teams advances the assets of local human resources. Team members who work cooperatively, and share information and duties about patients, learn multitasking skills to cover different areas of expertise in patient care; the effect is a reduction

of gaps in care that can impact the management of complex patients and reduce the quality of support (Lazzari, Shoka, Papanna and Kulkarni, 2018).

MRT 2
Person-centred care for patients with health conditions can be maintained as long as each interprofessional team member can address patients' multiple needs in a multitasking fashion. Person-centred care can (only) develop in the networks of relationship interplays of carers within themselves, carers with patients, carers with families and families with patients (Lazzari, Shoka, Papanna and Mousalidis, 2017). In other words, person-centred care is structured on systemic networks of interactions and team communication where patients are part participants in their recovery (Lazzari, Shoka, Papanna and Mousalidis, 2017) (Figure 3.6.).

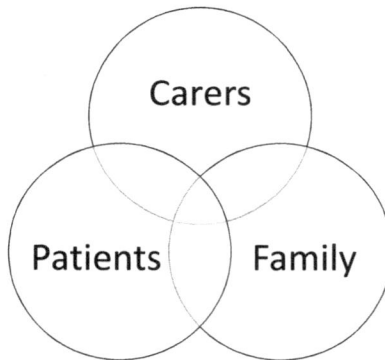

Figure 3.6. – Patient-centred care is the family, patients and carers integrated system network.

MRT 3
Suppose team members can adapt their skills to cover multiple areas of patients' needs and have their colleagues' support. In that case, patient-centred care, high patient safety and healthcare quality are feasible (Lazzari and Shoka, 2016). Coordinating with colleagues from multiple areas of expertise improves the corporate management of complex cases, such as patients or families, when they are unhappy with the services

and care provided (Lazzari and Shoka, 2016). Interprofessional systems can change dynamically whenever team members can perform different tasks (e.g., a nurse being matron and helping in physical check-ups) within the organisation and when new members arrive and can change the team's setup (Johnson, 2019).

MRT 4
SNA can help extract the network configuration of task distribution in healthcare settings (Lazzari, 2019). Likely, several healthcare settings will reflect the design of the unitasking versus multitasking distribution of healthcare labour when addressing patients' multiple needs (Lazzari, 2019).

MRT 5
The divide between those multitasker HCPs who want to go the extra mile and support patients in each aspect and those who, instead, remain in their area of expertise is likely to widen the fork of labour distribution and favour the careers and promotions of the multitaskers of their organisation; these last, at any moment, know how to respond to multiple patients' needs and handle the complexity in work demands (Lazzari and Thomas, 2018a, 2018b). Moreover, the team members we approached during our research felt that collateral support from colleagues is essential to reduce grief and burnout from attending to severely ill patients, workload and sharing duties for caring for complex cases (Lazzari and Thomas, 2018a, 2018b).

Our reflection *on* action, professional growth and a way to change

The unobtrusive ethnographic observation of who is doing what in hospital wards showed how unitasking and multitasking could hinder or promote integrated care for patients, synchronously or asynchronously. While some team members focused on a single aspect of patient care, others were multitaskers. We believe clinical governance should instead encourage 'each' member of the HCP team to be ready to attend to a patient's basic needs and, if the professional regulatory body allows, offer adequate support and bridge training for other areas of expertise. We usually cover our medical, professional or pedagogical role but also help in other areas of expertise that belong to our colleagues, supporting them in their activities as long as this action is regulated and does not breach our professional obligations. Therefore, integrated care means that each team member can address multiple patients' needs independently from their professional role and is willing to move from unitasking to multitasking.

The next stage of the research

If, in this chapter, we looked at the distribution of labour within interprofessional teams according to the work that needs to be done, in the following one, it was necessary to capture interprofessional teams' central figures in knowledge management and information gatekeepers. To our knowledge, the methodological approach of the subsequent study complements the current chapter as it captures the configuration of interprofessional teams in healthcare organisations, measures the degree of interpersonal links and illustrates the magnitude of the centrality of specific HCPs according to their area of specialisation. This approach is novel and has never been applied in the study of interprofessional teams (Figure 3.7.).

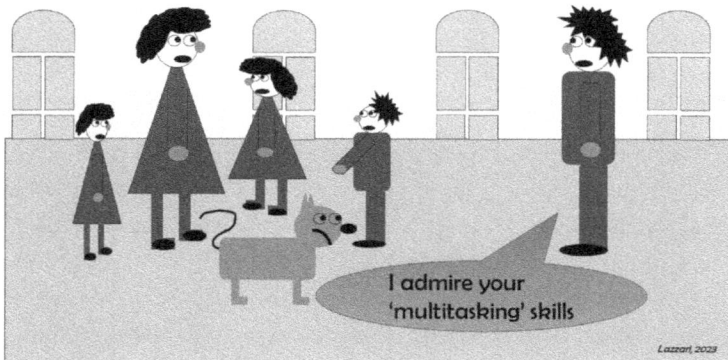

Figure 3.7. – Multitasking should be a plus in interprofessional teams and not a diverted responsibility of unitasking professionals from their duties.

CHAPTER 4

Teamwork and Collaboration

Abstract

The current chapter extracts the salient theoretical and practical aspects of interprofessional practice. The supporting publication is Lazzari, C., Kotera, Y., Green, P. and Rabottini, M. (2021) 'Social network analysis of Alzheimer's teams: A clinical review and applications in psychiatry to explore interprofessional care', *Current Alzheimer Research*, 18(5): pp. 380–398. The study supplied important insight into interprofessional practice using robust instruments to map interprofessional links and measure their intensity.

Our reflection *in* action

The following passage is a quote from our chronicle, which we kept when we conducted this study and worked in interprofessional teams. The excerpt encapsulates the issue that prompted our research question and the writing of this chapter. It is an ad verbatim extraction of our conversation with colleagues in healthcare settings.

> «It does not matter if we work asynchronously, at different times and shifts on the same goal, or synchronously, all simultaneously; there appear to be gaps in our team regarding the division of labour and accountability, while communication exchanges favour some and hinder others. We feel we also have the professional obligation to provide

our input to the team because we are in a high-ranking position. Yet, we often find that professionals from the same educational background (e.g., nurses with nurses, social workers with social workers) do not frequently liaise with other team members from different educational experiences (e.g., nurses with doctors). We believe that *intra*-professional (within the same area of expertise) communication links create bottlenecks in information sharing compared to *inter*-professional (within different areas of expertise). This configuration might create the premises for reduced information and knowledge-sharing within interprofessional teams. The needed information is not well circulated among all team members to provide unitary care. We want to study this aspect and have statistical confirmation» (Table 4.1.).

Table 4.1. – Reflection in action in teamwork and strategies.

The actual event	Considering it when it was occurring	Settings where applied	Acting without delay (motto)	Choosing how to respond at the moment
Intraprofessional bottleneck.	Some team members engage solely with others from the same educational or high-ranking backgrounds (e.g., a high-ranking nurse with a junior nurse) and might undervalue the contribution of others in the same area of expertise.	Daily routines within a team, handovers, MDT meetings.	Evaluate and prize each one in your team.	Team leaders, high-rankings, and ward managers ensure immediate engagement and communication when they see that some professional figures have been overlooked or have not provided input in patient care.

The actual event	Considering it when it was occurring	Settings where applied	Acting without delay (motto)	Choosing how to respond at the moment
Interprofessional bottleneck.	Some team members engage solely with others from the same level of seniority and expertise (e.g., a high-ranking nurse with a high-ranking doctor) and might undervalue the contribution of co-workers from other areas of expertise.	Ibid.	Discussion means contribution.	The team leader explores each participant's contribution to the team discussion, ensuring that all participants representing different areas of expertise are included in the global patient discussions.

Background

This chapter was developed from the two previous studies. We used the following analytic question to understand how interprofessional teams in healthcare are configured and the dimensions of the interprofessional links: What are the characteristics of interprofessional practice? Who is occupying the most central positions in knowledge management and information flow? (see Overholser, 1993; Carona, Handford and Fonseca, 2021). The study aimed to determine whether we could measure the intensity of the bonds between interprofessional team members and whether we could capture such teams' configurations and discover their central players.

Our early analysis of teamwork in healthcare organisations revealed that when the team members used prevalent intra-professional (within the same professional role) information sharing and communication—the primary goals of collaborative care—the patient care goals of the organisation were not always met (Lazzari, 1998). New communicative strategies were thus needed to implement interprofessional communication (Lazzari, Masiello and Shoka, 2017).

According to Argyris and Schön (1996), learning involves finding and correcting problems. In our setting, 'single-loop learning' ensues when a job-related difficulty is detected and addressed to enable the organisation to continue its present policies or attain its current objectives

(Argyris and Schön, 1996). Alternatively, 'double-loop learning' occurs when an organisation's fundamental rules, policies and methods may be modified to identify and correct issues (Argyris and Schön, 1996). We thus asked ourselves what the 'problem' we wanted to find evidence for was and that we tried to solve by proposing policies. We thus answered: better quality of care from the interprofessional practice.

Interprofessional healthcare teams focus on patients. Successful patient care occurs when interprofessional team members effectively share their care plans and knowledge capital, regardless of their speciality areas (Lazzari and Masino, 2015). Patients, too, are sensitive to how their allocated healthcare team members—nurses, social workers, doctors and others—treat them, entrusting them to be reliable and coordinated in their communal efforts (e.g., sharing information and care between primary and secondary organisations). This process alerts patients to any incongruence and gaps in their care teams, for instance, when the cooperating carers appear split in the patient's care plans (Lazzari and Masino, 2015).

This is why coordinated care is registered as satisfactory or unsatisfactory from the patients' side. To merge HCP's efforts, interprofessional teams rely on the advice of a few central and high-ranking members of the group, who are the champions in information management (Lazzari, Kotera, Green and Rabottini, 2021). However, the intense centralisation of knowledge and data administration in healthcare teams might also marginalise other professionals who can equally convey critical information in patient care (Lazzari, Kotera, Green and Rabottini, 2021). Sometimes, interprofessional teams might underestimate the contribution of some HCPs who might not be in high-ranking positions in the medical and nursing specialities or work remotely or part-time in the hospital, ward or organisation (Lazzari, Kotera, Green and Rabottini, 2021). The risk is that their information and knowledge capital in strategic decision-making regarding patient care, assessment and intervention might not be acknowledged (Lazzari, Kotera, Green and Rabottini, 2021; Figure 4.1).

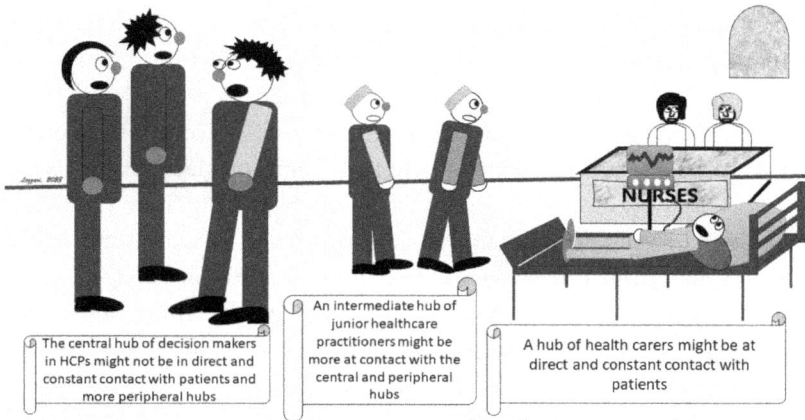

Figure 4.1. – Several small groups of professionals in an extended social network. Those in the central position are usually the significant decision-makers, although important information can also be at the network's periphery.

Wanting to fill gaps in healthcare settings, we will look at how to optimise interprofessional teamwork and promote the democratic participation of all team members. In the 1960s and 1970s, there was the beginning of a movement where the public requested greater liability by healthcare organisations and their expenses, prompting evidence-based research with a desire to determine whether or not governmental grants were wisely used to accomplish policy objectives (Yanow, 2018). More legislators with a medical background are now gravitating towards quality and safety improvement, in which care delivery systems are carefully examined for errors and breakdowns, focusing on how multi-professional groups strive to make the necessary improvements (Zwarenstein and Reeves, 2006). According to the Royal College of Physicians, incidents of professional negligence commonly arise when interprofessional teams fail to cooperate effectively with one another and share information (Germain, 2001).

Case scenario

Once, one of the authors (CL) worked in a psychiatric hospital for children (CAHMS). He was concerned about an adolescent girl who was an inpatient with autism and a personality disorder. It was winter, and she had turned the heater off in her room and opened the windows, exposing herself to the risk of a chest infection. At first, no team member knew this; only an allied healthcare professional, who constantly supervised the girl, knew. Although this worker shared his notes with the other staff members through common electronic records, since he did not have a 'central and more high-ranking' role, the other team members underestimated the information he constantly gave them about the girl's behaviour. But when the author (at that time, one of the new senior team members) read his electronic notes and saw the girl for the first time, he realised that the report was critical and the girl's behaviour risky. So, he immediately took action to help the girl and improve her health. This chapter illustrates this process of centralisation and periphery in the social networks of interprofessional teams. Conducting this research, we grew as professionals, realising that the input of any team member in multidisciplinary teams is vital for achieving effective care and reducing the risks patients pose to themselves and others.

Methods used

Our approach to analysis has been inspired by Margaret Mead's anthropological method, which avoids the observer's bias when utilising checklists by identifying the traits of the detected behaviour (Mead, 1977). Hence, we adopted adequate evaluation techniques to capture the nature and extent of interprofessional activity using statistical tools (SNA and quantitative approaches); we aimed to measure the degree of collaborative care (Lazzari and Rabottini, 2021). Social Network Analysis (SNA) may also appraise team dynamics, knowledge-sharing within networks, and organisational connections. It can also provide suggestions for improving care safety and patient treatment value (Cunningham et al., 2012). For instance, SNA explores how one individual or entity exchanges ideas, assets and information with others (Crossley et al., 2015). SNA may also assist in identifying spheres for development in interprofessional treatment and can visually depict the hidden relationships among network players (Cross and Parker, 2004;

Lockhart, 2017). As a result, SNA is a frame of mixed-method enquiry that demonstrates that social events include transactions, connections and agreements that link one actor (e.g., person) or node to another actor or node and that aid in determining the statistical significance of the arrangement of these relationships (Scott, 2017).

The elements of a social network are called 'nodes' or 'actors', which stand in for people or organisations, and 'ties', 'edges' or 'arrows', which indicate the relationships between the nodes (Prell, 2012; Yang et al., 2017). Double-headed arrows indicate higher and reciprocal collaboration between the elements of a social network and designate the mutual exchange of information or resources and interactions between nodes or players; the opposite occurs with one-headed arrows indicating unilateral interactions (Yang et al., 2017; Figure 4.2).

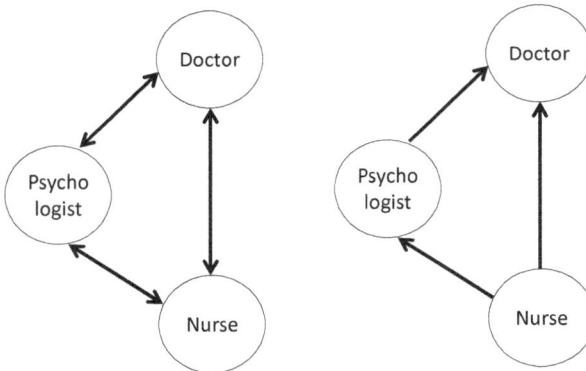

Figure 4.2. – Examples of reciprocal (left) and unilateral (right) social ties and communication within networks or HCPs (Lazzari et al., 2021).

The principle of SNA holds that all units are interconnected, and changes in one unit impact other units (Tsvetovat and Kouznetosov, 2011). Additionally, 'centrality' in a network denotes when a person or node has a lot of both internal and external connections, while 'prestige' is the case when incoming ties predominate; a centrality score of 100% denotes that a person has links with everyone else in the network (Knoke and Yang, 2008; Prell, 2012). If the study found the degree of centrality to be higher in some nodes or actors, we could assume that they were probably the information gatekeepers in the network studied.

Social systems can be explained using Wiener's theory, which demonstrates the similarities between neurological and societal organisations (Wiener, 2013). When he saw people with neurological impairments, he concluded that to interact with the world appropriately, not only do we need an efficient registration of signals from the world—for example, the neurological process of a heat source—but these signals must go back to the central nervous system to combine this information with other information coming from different senses to produce an adequate response to the neurological signals—for example, muscular contraction to avoid pain (Wiener, 2013). We adopted these concepts to extract the MRTs from this study.

Findings

Consultants, mid-level physicians, specialist registrars or associate specialists, junior physicians or residents, ward managers, nurses, sisters, clinical leaders, healthcare assistants, psychologists, occupational therapists, social workers, hospital administrators and ward pharmacists were all part of the teams' intended clientele. Considering that a 100% 'degree of prestige' in SNA means that an HCP is 'the centre' of all information flow, the outcomes of this study established that some HCPs occupied central positions in the social network with a high % of centralities, such as the consultant (21.37%), ward manager (16.55%), high-ranking nurse (16.55%), speciality doctor (11%) and registered nurse (8.96%) (Lazzari et al., 2021). However, not all interactions were symmetrical in reciprocal interchanges of information and advice, as a high degree of centrality did not mean that the information was mutual (double-headed arrows), indicating a higher degree of incoming (receiving advice from the team) or outgoing (providing advice to the team) flow of information but not both (Lazzari et al., 2021). Instead, in SNA, the parameter to measure reciprocity in communication flow is called r, with a value of 1.0 indicating a person's reciprocal exchange of information with any other team member (Scott, 2017). The study found that clinical psychologists had the most symmetric relationships with other professions, followed by occupational therapists, social workers, student nurses, healthcare assistants, middle-grade physicians and junior physicians (Lazzari et al., 2021).

Discussions and middle-range theories

We found that the most high-ranking persons in HCPs were at the pivot of decision-making and advice-giving; however, not all information exchanges they promoted were two-way (Lazzari et al., 2021). Some HCPs occupied more peripheral positions in the information network, as their knowledge and data did not frequently reach the central decision hubs (Lazzari, 2019b; Lazzari et al., 2021). The derived configuration demonstrated a significant hub of high-ranking practitioners more regularly communicating with each other–usually, high-ranking nurses and doctors or professionals from the same educational background. The periphery of the network was instead occupied by junior positions till the boundary, which was engaged by the other HCPs such as community nurses or social workers, whose impact on the information flow and knowledge management in patient care, from time to time, resulted somehow marginal, especially when patients were hospitalised and away from their home (Lazzari et al., 2021; Figures 4.3. and 4.4.).

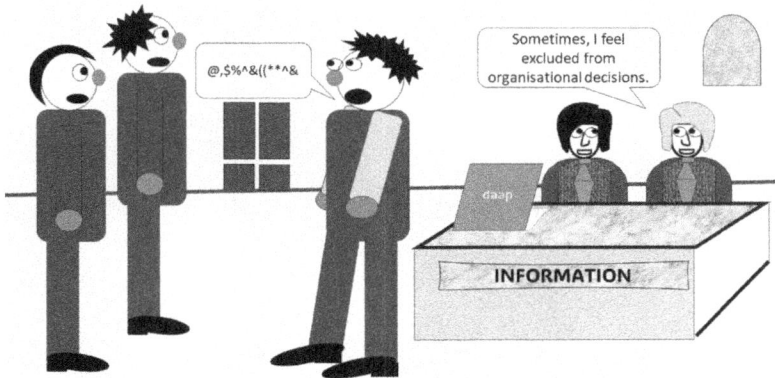

Figure 4.3. – Feeling that their information might not be included in the team's decisions could generate frustration and reduce the psychological contract of some team members with the organisation.

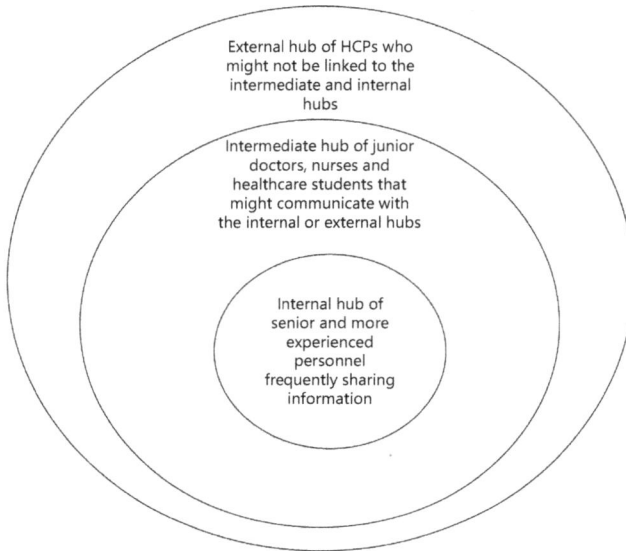

Figure 4.4. – The social network of interprofessional teams in hospital wards sees the high degree of centrality of high-ranking professionals, such as consultants, ward managers, geriatric nurses, middle-grade doctors and registered nurses. They are often the information gatekeepers, manage the information flow to the rest of the team, provide advice on patient care and receive the necessary information from team members to decide on care plans. However, with progressive social distance from the central hubs, some HCPs might not impact the central decisional hub, and their information and wealth of data regarding patients might be underestimated.

Middle-range theories

We extracted the following MRTs from the current study as corroborated and developed from our previous research.

MRT 1

An organisational social system's ability to achieve its objectives and maintain its vitality and functionality is analogous to that of a biological system, as both the members of the system and the environment benefit from a two-way flow of information and knowledge that is provided via feedback mechanisms (Lazzari and Masiello, 2016).

MRT 2

The network analysis of healthcare interprofessional teamwork revealed bottlenecks in information sharing and knowledge management due to the centralisation of information and data sharing, sometimes privileging more high-ranking or experienced professionals (Lazzari, Masiello and Shoka, 2017). Owing to the network or social distance from the central gatekeepers in clinical information, other junior professionals and those who might not cover central (and pivotal) medical and nursing roles risk losing their wealth of data; their knowledge capital might not be shared within the whole team (Lazzari and Thomas, 2018).

MRT 3

Interprofessional communication can be verbal, written or visual; it can be synchronous when the exchange occurs through face-to-face encounters or asynchronous through, for example, electronic, digital and analogic clinical records or emails. Each piece of information is vital to patient care. In addition, any team member can hold essential bits of information; integrated care supports the democratic sharing of individual (patients') data holistically (Lazzari, McAleer and Rabottini, 2021). The divide between the central hubs of HCPs who share information more intensely and frequently (among them) and the peripheral hubs of HCPs who are outside the main information flow might risk creating information gaps, information bottlenecks and broken communication links that could harm the patients' and carers' health and safety (Lazzari, Kotera and Thomas, 2019).

Our reflections *on* the action, professional growth and a way to change

From our experience with teams, we realised that some HCPs were champions in information sharing and providing and receiving advice on patient care while delegating information to others in the group to get the job done. We learned to do the same. When we conduct a multidisciplinary team (MDT), we endeavour to involve all our team members, for instance, via Microsoft Teams, Zoom and other online platforms if they cannot attend in person. We have grown professionally as high-ranking practitioners in hospitals and academia in the UK. We feel confident in making recommendations for interprofessional practice by encouraging every team member to share their knowledge and information about patients and service users of the team (e.g., students) with others. We also encourage high-ranking members to listen to the information junior professionals and students want to share. We now work in universities and healthcare settings. Our role and responsibilities dictate that we coordinate the efforts of our group of skilful health practitioners and academic teachers. We like it when everyone in interprofessional teams takes their duties seriously, and clinical or academic information is shared with others to integrate assessments, care plans, educational projects and any goal the team should achieve. Moreover, verbal and non-verbal behaviour skill is necessary for successful teamwork (Figure 4.5).

The next stage of the research

After completing this chapter, we had sufficient elements to create a tailored interprofessional education to improve the skills of undergraduate healthcare professionals for delivering improved, coordinated and effective patient care. Hence, the following chapter condenses the pedagogical aspects of interprofessional practice while highlighting the factors that favour or hinder learning collaborative relationships. This was also the first study where mobile and smartphone technology assessed and promoted interprofessional learning in healthcare students.

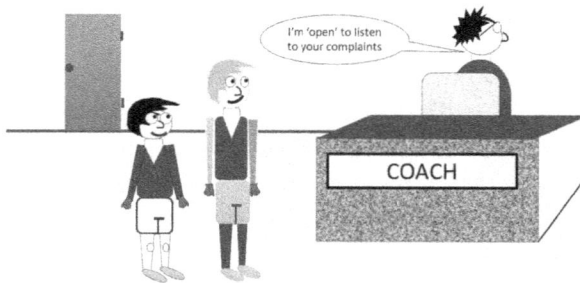

Lazzari, 2023

Figure 4.5. – Non-verbal communication in interprofessional teams is a powerful tool that stabilises or undermines the whole team.

CHAPTER 5

Learning Interprofessional Practice

Abstract

The current chapter extracts the salient theoretical and practical aspects of interprofessional education. The supporting publication is Lazzari, C., McAleer, S., Nusair, A. and Rabottini, M. (2021) 'Psychiatric training during COVID-19 pandemic benefits from integrated practice in interprofessional teams and ecological momentary e-assessment', *Rivista di Psichiatria*, 56(2), pp. 74–84. We explore pedagogical assessments in real-time (EMA: Ecologic Momentary Assessment) and extract modern pedagogical theories in learning and interprofessional education. As emphasised in the section, the reinforcement of learners' mindfulness of teamwork directly affects their academic fulfilment, confidence in their clinical skills and the quality of care.

Our reflection *in* action

The following section is an extract from our diary, which we kept when we conducted this study and worked in interprofessional and interdisciplinary teams. This extract encapsulates the issue that prompted our research question and the writing of this chapter. It is an ad verbatim extraction of our conversation with our colleagues about starting a research project on interprofessional education (June 2018):

> «We are interested in studying and promoting interprofessional education. We participate in multi-professional teams

every day. We notice how the quality of our interactions affects our work and job satisfaction. We read about the new development of educational technology and smartphones to access and promote students' progress in a real-time and actual scenario. It is an 'ecological momentary assessment'. We believe it is a good idea to use smartphone technology as a formative assessment of interprofessional education as we can have the continuing outcomes of our programmes and learners' progress in the actual settings where they operate. We are also interested in new pedagogical theories that emphasise the impact of learners' emotions on their interprofessional learning and progression. We read about 'flow psychology' and want to apply it to interprofessional education. The outcomes will attract health carers, medical teachers and healthcare policymakers as we reflect on what is new in the pedagogical assessment of interprofessional practice» (Table 5.1).

Table 5.1. – Reflection in action in teamwork and strategies

The actual event	Considering it when it was occurring	Settings where applied	Acting without delay (motto)	Choosing how to respond at the moment
Interprofessional learning in medical and nursing schools.	Learning interprofessional practice.	Team discussion of patients and bedside assessments and treatments.	Learn with, from, and about others.	Learners of interprofessional courses discover to ask for support from mates from other areas of expertise to engage successfully with patients.
Ibid.	Accessing a survey to appraise the own progress.	Ibid.	Become self-reflective on your relationships with others.	Learners use skills to monitor their emotions in working in teams and regulate their resilience during collective participation.

Background

An intervention known as interprofessional education (IPE) is one in which students from diverse health or social care professions learn how to cooperate to advance their skills in collaborative care with the declared objectives of improving patient/client health/wellness or both and interpersonal skills (Reeves et al., 2018).

IPE prepares students for health professions where cooperation and teamwork are crucial (van Diggele et al., 2020). International health organisations have pushed IPE to improve interprofessional collaboration, patient care and public health (Lazzari, 2019a). As a result, universities have begun developing and maintaining comprehensive and authentic IPE programmes for healthcare students (van Diggele et al., 2020). Self-reflection is one major route for IPE learners to understand their sense of self and what happens when interacting with others (Lazzari and Masiello, 2017a). Self-reflection is crucial for IPE learning (Lazzari and Masiello, 2017b).

Other authors have also employed knowledge and understanding, self-reflection and collective mindfulness questions throughout IPE (Olson et al., 2016). Self-reflection fosters empathy and compassion and the investigation of one's cultural lenses, cultural distinctions among classmates and the socio-emotional challenges associated with delivering culturally responsive care (Olson et al., 2016). Mobile technology (e.g., smartphones and the Internet) to assess learners' progress and ongoing emotions and outcomes can promote a self-reflective practice; this process is called ecological momentary assessment (Willet et al., 2012). Learners' mindfulness often matches self-reflection on their state of mind and thoughts (Black and William, 2008).

Additionally, there is a connection between mindfulness and learning: students who self-evaluate their performance do better than those who do not (Andrade and Valtcheva, 2009). In pursuing an educational approach to interprofessional training, we were influenced by the theory of Mihaly Csikszentmihalyi's *flow psychology* in education. As Csikszentmihalyi explains, deep concentration becomes action and awareness, which, in turn, become feelings of control, making the person forget the efforts in the task; such engagement leads to a sense of spontaneity and effortless behaviour (cited in Beard, 2015). Feelings of *flow* occur when our psychological energy and attention are engaged in achievable goals, and we feel that we have the skills to reach those goals (Csikszentmihalyi, 1990).

Being constantly mindful of ourselves and focused on our activity is central to the flow experience; at such a mindful moment, we momentarily disregard everything else, with only our pursuit of our goal directing our consciousness (Csikszentmihalyi, 1990). To achieve an optimal learning experience, learners use an 'autotelic' attitude, meaning that they will pursue an action for its satisfaction; at the same time, the flow will flourish if a person can balance curiosity and match it with the skills to master an experience (Tarling, 2016). For example, suppose learners perceive that they are curious about achieving a specific goal but recognise that they lack sufficient skills to attain the desired destination; in this case, not flow but frustration ensues (Tarling, 2016).

Csikszentmihalyi (1997) compares the joy of an optimal learning activity to that demonstrated by students in art schools, stating that aesthetic actions augment the quality of continuous experience in a way that few others do. Suppose that individuals perceive that they can dynamically interact with their social and physical environment and feel resourceful in interpreting and addressing the demands of that environment; in this case, flow ensues (Schermuly and Meyer, 2020). For instance, sometimes we felt reduced personal satisfaction and feelings of mastery—and thus flow—when we were assigned simple administrative work (i.e. typing letters). At the same time, we thought we could be better employed in complex clinical and academic jobs (e.g., assessing and treating difficult patients or reviewing dissertations). As Csikszentmihalyi (1997) suggests, the merging of students' skills and academic challenges results in nine academic emotions: (1) worry, which derives from the combination of a moderate challenge and low skills; (2) anxiety, which derives from the combination of a high challenge and low skills; (3) arousal, which derives from the combination of a high challenge and moderate skills; (4) flow, which derives from the combination of a high challenge and high skills; (5) control, which derives from the combination of a moderate challenge and high skills; (6) boredom, which derives from the combination of a low challenge and high skills; (7) relaxation, which derives from the combination of a low challenge and moderate skills; and (8) apathy, which derives from the combination of a low challenge and low skills (Figure 5.1.).

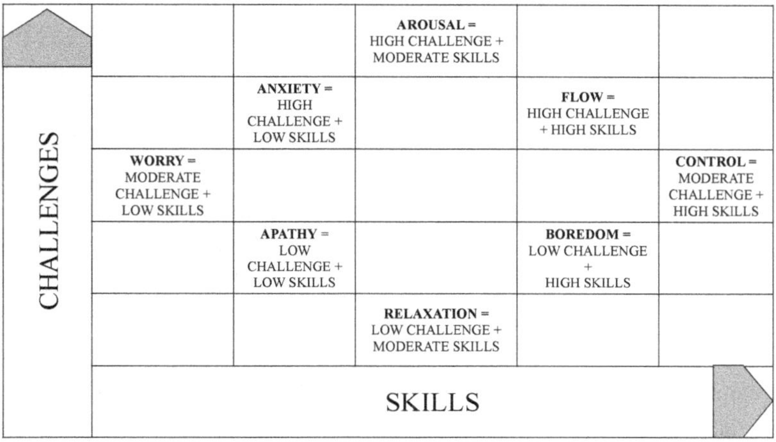

CHALLENGES			AROUSAL = HIGH CHALLENGE + MODERATE SKILLS		
		ANXIETY = HIGH CHALLENGE + LOW SKILLS		FLOW = HIGH CHALLENGE + HIGH SKILLS	
	WORRY = MODERATE CHALLENGE + LOW SKILLS				CONTROL = MODERATE CHALLENGE + HIGH SKILLS
		APATHY = LOW CHALLENGE + LOW SKILLS		BOREDOM = LOW CHALLENGE + HIGH SKILLS	
			RELAXATION = LOW CHALLENGE + MODERATE SKILLS		
			SKILLS		

Figure 5.1. – Academic emotions derive from matching academic challenges with students' skills to cope with these challenges (see Csikszentmihalyi, 1997).

The value of learning in interprofessional practice is not only linked to emotional experiences, as in Csikszentmihalyi, but is also associated with an ethical endeavour of learning mutual respect and physical resistance to social and interpersonal stress from working in hectic teams (for instance, hospital emergency departments) (Lazzari and Masiello, 2017b).

Two theories connected to emotional intelligence were pioneered by the Milan School model of the eight channels (Delle Fave and Massimi, 2005; Delle Fave, Massimi and Bassi, 2011). According to the Milan School, when students encounter problems and overcome them using abilities slightly beyond their customary norms, they sense self-mastery and engage in productive learning (Delle Fave and Massimi, 2005; Delle Fave, Massimi and Bassi, 2011).

Learning and kalokagathia

According to the Ancient Greeks, moral ideals in education were referred to as *Kalokagathia*, indicating the beauty and gallantry of a human being (Bazaluk, 2017). *Kalokagathia* is made from *Kalos* and *Agathos*: the former signifies 'beautiful', indicating to each Greek that the primary aim of education should be to attain an object or goal that is aesthetically beautiful; the latter signifies 'worthy' or 'good' in the knightly sense, thus illustrating the purpose and moral values of education (Bazaluk, 2017)[1]. The two concepts are strictly linked in WBL and, therefore, in interprofessional practice. Team members aim to reach the *Kalos*, a pleasant and appealing job, not being overwhelmed by stress to work efficiently in teams and not be overwhelmed by the fatigue and frustration of interpersonal relationship demands (Lazzari and Shoka, 2016). Having emotional and physical resilience will help the team focus more on job demands without feeling exhausted while interacting efficiently in interprofessional teams, perceiving that no member is trespassing on norms of mutual and moral respect or *Agathos* (Lazzari, Shoka and Masiello, 2016).

Similarly, ensuring mutual respect will help interprofessional relationships and collaborative care by boosting personnel morale. At the same time, team members' WBL is the achievement of moral values to treat others in the group and patients justly and respectfully—that is, with *Agathos* (Thomas and Mousailidis, 2017). To become ethically minded in interprofessional practice and address their own and others' needs for fair and shared participation in their approach, healthcare learners and HCPs must become self-reflective and assess where they are on their learning pathways and moral development (Lazzari, Shoka, Papanna and Mousailidis, 2017). They must endure the constant stress

1 The etymological meaning of *school*: [place of instruction] Middle English scole, from Old English scol, 'institution for instruction,' from Latin schola 'meeting place for teachers and students, place of instruction;' also 'learned conversation, debate; lecture; disciples of a teacher, body of followers, sect,' also in the older Greek skholē 'spare time, leisure, rest, ease; idleness; that in which leisure is employed; learned discussion;' sense of 'intermission of work, leisure for learning.' [Reference: www.etymonline.com. (n.d.). *school | Origin and meaning of school by Online Etymology Dictionary*. [online] Available at: https://www.etymonline.com/word/school].

in interprofessional conflicts, focus on their goals, be mindful of their limitations and believe they have the skills to achieve them; this last is particularly important to deal with challenging patients and colleagues (Lazzari, Shoka, Papanna and Mousailidis, 2017).

Self-reflective practice

The self-reflective practice in learning is drawn from the idea of 'reflection-as-action', whereby pondering one's understanding serves as the foundation of education (Bleakley, 1999; Hébert, 2015). According to Bleakley (1999), a reflective practice encourages students to be conscious and build their capacity for self-reflection. Furthermore, there is a link between mindfulness and learning: students who self-evaluate their performance are more successful than those who do not (Andrade and Valtcheva, 2009).

Students engage in 'reflection-in-action' when they can access a formative assessment during and immediately after their training; usually, self-reflective practice occurs while educational events are ongoing (Lazzari, 2018; Lazzari, McAleer, Nusair and Rabottini, 2021). Learners can participate in 'reflection-on-action' when self-appraisal occurs immediately after an educational event's conclusion (see Schön, 1987). Also, at this point, the learners face two aspects of their learning: pedagogical challenges, such as interprofessional tasks, and pedagogical skills, such as their attitude to deal with these challenges (Lazzari, McAleer, Nusair and Rabottini, 2021).

Methodological approach

We suggest that ecological momentary assessment (EMA) can continuously evaluate the attitudes and abilities of the learners. EMA measurements focus on information on a learner's transitory state, such as events that occur emotionally, cognitively and behaviourally shortly after a learning experience and that happen in the learner's usual context or a standard-situation environment (Stone and Shiffman, 1994; Stone, 2007; Shiffman, Stone and Hufford, 2008). The EMA reported in one of our studies was comprehensive when students used electronic, online platforms and devices (EMeA) to access the relevant surveys, questionnaires or evaluation tools while still participating in their clinical scenario and learning task as an interprofessional team.

This ongoing real-time evaluation reduced recollection bias and gave researchers a better grasp of how healthcare students interact with one another (Stone, 2007; Shiffman et al., 2008; Goodwin, Velicer and Intille, 2008; Yoshiuchi, Yamamoto and Akabayashi, 2008; Willet et al., 2012; Moskowitz and Young, 2006). Additionally, EMA enables medical teachers to modify an ongoing clinical programme and inform students of the areas that need reinforcement, providing immediate feedback to medical and nursing students (Ellaway and Master, 2008; Maudsley et al., 2018). According to a systematic study, medical students may utilise mobile technology, such as cell phones, to record their instructors' evaluations in clinical settings and track their skill growth (Ellaway and Master, 2008; Maudsley et al., 2018).

Findings

As *flow education* is paramount, students and mentors participating in our study agreed to face interprofessional challenges that did not exceed the students' feelings of competence. They did not affect their emotional well-being by creating anxiety, worry, apathy or boredom. The study that supports the current chapter surveyed undergraduate students in interprofessional training for two weeks, including student nurses, doctors, and occupational therapists. According to the study outcomes, 59% felt that the academic challenges met their target standards and that they had the skills to meet them. The most prevailing *flow* of *educational* emotions in IPE was relaxation in 58% of learners, feeling in control in 30%, feeling excited in 10%, feeling happy (flow) in 13% and feeling glad in 20%. In comparison, 8% felt bored, 15% anxious, and 8% worried. About 60% felt satisfied to very satisfied with the interprofessional education.

The importance of emphasising academic feelings and nurturing pleasant emotions, enjoyment and gratification in the learners aligns with Knowles's andragogy ideologies, which state that an education setting should reassure, trust and respect pupils (Melick and Melick, 2010). The study's findings also give credence to van Manen's (2010) thesis, which holds that students learn more effectively and become self-reflective when collaborating with peers on activities and skills through feeling the self and others, known as 'pathic knowledge' (van Manen, 2010). This last refers to personal mindfulness about being in a relationship with others, the settings, and the routines and practices at a pre-cognitive or meta-cognitive level (van Manen, 2010). Therefore, although 58% of students thought interprofessional learning was a low-level difficulty, they all believed they possessed the necessary teamwork abilities. Comparatively, 30% of participants perceived interprofessional practice as challenging even if they had intermediate teamwork abilities.

Moreover, emerging from this study, the students recognised the value of sharing care plans and engaging in interprofessional communication to enhance their collaborative practice. Small-scale groups made it easier for people to work together and solve problems (Fraser, 2001). In our observations, people (and interprofessional students) could learn new behavioural models by being exposed to them directly or seeing how others acted (Bandura, 1971). The students who used their cell phones for ongoing e-assessment throughout the described study also showed more sensitivity to interprofessional occurrences and a propensity for future interprofessional teamwork. This outcome lends credibility to the idea that (self-)assessing students—in this case, through online technology—often encourages critical thinking, self-awareness and observation (Malthouse, Watts and Roffer-Barnsten, 2015).

Group learning changes into shared understanding when students behave increasingly as a collaborating system, interacting with a sense of communal involvement and assistance and conveying patient data, choices and strategies for treating their patients (see Mezirow, 1997). Students also said that patients could identify when an interprofessional team was treating them. Healthcare customers acknowledged the value of getting treatment from a coordinated staff and interprofessional teamwork (Lazzari, McAleer, Nusair and Rabottini 2021). In the case of cooperative care, customers' satisfaction and the level of care were optimal (Lazzari, McAleer, Nusair and Rabottini 2021). We also found that, after learning interprofessional skills, learners could realise that cooperation could run smoothly and that the whole team could easily reach its shared care target (Lazzari, McAleer, Nusair and Rabottini 2021). Furthermore, successful cooperative care was ensured when each learner discovered how to be courteous, empathic, humble, credible, transparent and skilful when working with their colleagues (Lazzari, McAleer, Nusair and Rabottini 2021). Positive interpersonal skills also had a positive cascade outcome on the excellence of care, resulting in constructive patient feedback and reaching the clinical target set by the interprofessional team and organisation (Lazzari, McAleer, Nusair and Rabottini, 2021).

WBL learning and middle-range theories (MRTs)

The following are the MRTs extractable from the current chapter and study, complementing our previous research on the topic.

MRT-1

Interprofessional education (IPE) can be encouraged by improving flow experiences among students. Medical teachers should bring learners before challenges slightly above their standards while ensuring they have sufficient skills to progress to their next developmental stage (Lazzari and Masiello, 2017a).

MRT-2

Interprofessional practice can promote mutual respect and empathy when learners are aware of their flow experiences and mindful of their emotions during team interactions (Lazzari and Masiello, 2017a). Improving interprofessional practice has the beneficial effects of fostering job satisfaction and patient appreciation in integrated healthcare while enhancing patient care outcomes (Lazzari and Masiello, 2017b).

MRT-3

Changes in interprofessional practice are dynamic, and a constant feedback mechanism from learners to mentors/organisations/teachers and vice versa can provide a real-time grasp of the ongoing learners' interprofessional emotions, learning, flow and needs (Lazzari and Masiello, 2017b). Doing so will also facilitate integrated care plans in systemically oriented healthcare organisations and improve patient welfare and the value of care (Lazzari and Masiello, 2017c).

Conclusions

This chapter reinforces the importance of new pedagogical perspectives in interprofessional learning. Mezirow (2003) defined *transformative learning* as the knowledge that alters dysfunctional and biased ideas— sets of established expectations and misconceptions (habits of mind, understanding, attitudes, mentalities)—to open them up, making them more reflective, comprehensive, informed and psychologically malleable. Preconceived notions comprise rigid relational conceptions, ideologies, dogmatic orientation, stereotyped attitudes and behaviours, mental models for work, religious beliefs, moral-ethical standards, psychological preferences and schema, scientific and mathematical paradigms, linguistic and social science frameworks, and aesthetic ideals and standards (Mezirow, 2013). Critical analysis of the inferences that support our understandings, viewpoints, perspectives and mental models, as put out by Mezirow (1997), affects our frames of reference.

The current chapter's findings are consistent with Mezirow's (2003) model of *transformative learning*, in which apprentices who participate in a communal endeavour of creating and internalising a new or updated understanding of their experiences can alter their behaviour in the future to have less prejudiced ideas about other team members. In Mezirow's (2003) theory, transformational learning reappraises pre-existing beliefs and mindsets to include more comprehensive, unbiased, open, reflective mind frames for change. In contrast, fixed interpersonal relationships, conventional attitudes and routines, and vocational habits of thought are cognitive biases that reduce social learning (Mezirow, 2003). Therefore, corporate objectives could also be achieved by reinforcing ethical connections; learning rules of mutual respect and support between team members can strengthen their skills for sharing understanding and knowledge capital while improving customer relationships (Lazzari, 2004).

Our reflections *on* action, professional growth and a way to change

We could confirm that providing learners and HCPs with an environment conducive to implementing their sense of mastery and flow in teamwork can produce better patient care (Lazzari and Masiello, 2017c). Additionally, we aim to promote interprofessional care by focusing on the team's feelings of self-respect and appreciation of the roles of other team members from different professional backgrounds. We endeavour to encourage medical students, student nurses, any other healthcare professionals and ourselves to a sense of flow—that is, that level of pleasure achieved when we face challenges and use skills that could move us to the next level of learning while performing with feelings of mastery and joy (Lazzari and Masiello, 2017c).

In this sense, we would say that we can promote *kalokagathia* (the feeling of beauty and worth) through *flow* experiences and vice versa. By endorsing and promoting mutual respect in an interprofessional team, we might reinforce feelings of togetherness among team members and strengthen our work dedication and the psychological contract with our employer (Lazzari and Masiello, 2017b). We encourage policymakers and local team leaders to have reflective meetings to check if there are team members who need extra support and encouragement. Some HCPs might feel undermined or underestimated in their interprofessional practice. Instead, as the study shows, collaborating in a team requires applying skills of mutual understanding and respect independently from the clinical goals. This project also implies listening to the voices of those who are rarely heard. To conclude, this politic of inclusion has a positive cascade effect on patients, who can perceive whether an integrated and empathic team delivered their care. (Lazzari and Masiello, 2017a). Furthermore cooperative care boosts team members' job satisfaction and productivity as they feel involved in shared goals and respected by their teammates (Figure 5.2.).

The next stage of the research

At this point, we felt that our research had enough information about interprofessional practice. Our next step was to continue our research cycle and explore interprofessional-related concepts or co-occurring themes that emerge from the Web of Science. Moreover, we wanted to check whether other researchers had the same insights and reached the same conclusions as we did in our related research. According to our understanding, the following study is the first attempt to use bibliometric analysis to extract salient points in interprofessional practice from the Web of Science.

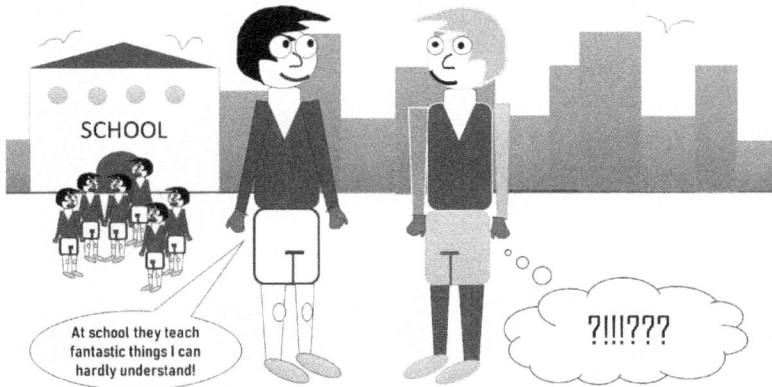

Figure 5.2. –Learners' emotions and skills are fundamental in creating and delivering educational material.

CHAPTER 6

Exploring the Existing Literature

Abstract

The current chapter extracts salient theories and observations from the study, Lazzari, C., McAleer, S. and Rabottini, M. (2022) 'The assessment of interprofessional practice in mental health nursing with ethnographic observation and social network analysis: A confirmatory and biblio-metric network study using VOSviewer', *Rivista di Psichiatria*, 57(3), pp. 115–122. It is time to focus on a broader range of interprofessional theories captured by the Web of Science. This step will help us endorse our observations and confirm what other authors have discovered in interprofessional practice.

Reflection *in* action

The following excerpt is from our journal, which we maintained when we conducted this study on interprofessional teams. It demonstrates the topic that sparked our research question and the writing of this chapter. It is a transcription of our discussion with our university colleagues about initiating a research project on interprofessional literature.

> «We want to conduct a study that tells us what the concepts involved are as extracted from the international literature in interprofessional practice. In the previous public works, we explored interprofessional teamwork as it exists in healthcare settings. We want to know how other researchers

approached the topic and what concepts they linked to cooperative healthcare. We thought that to confirm our finding, we need to take a step back and see what research, ideas and themes are related to 'interprofessional practice' emerging from the web of knowledge. If we can do this, we can validate and theoretically understand the topic we have treated».

Table 6.1. Reflection in action in teamwork and strategies.

The actual event	Considering it when it was occurring	Settings where applied	Acting without delay (motto)	Choosing how to respond at the moment
Exploring what other author authors are doing.	There is much research on interprofessional practice but limited reviews about how the central concepts are interrelated.	Web of Science (WoS) and interprofessional teams.	Know what interprofessional practice is and how it is applied.	Together with our team, we explore ways of interpreting collaborative practice which does not emerge from official documents and policies.
Understanding the underlying concepts.	The concepts and skills in interprofessional practice appear interlocked.	Ibid.	Thinking as a group includes the unity of our efforts and intent.	We are supported by other researchers that to work cooperatively, we need to share knowledge and leadership in our teams.

Theoretical background

This chapter aimed to understand the meanings of interprofessional practice. Epistemology is the study of knowledge (Encyclopaedia Britannica, 2022). Bloom's taxonomy of knowledge positions understanding meanings at the top of the pyramid (Budworth, Al Hashemi and Waddah, 2015). According to *Merriam-Webster Dictionary Online* (2021), 'meaning' is the idea defined by a term or expression. The first requirement is that all learning (inclusive interprofessional education) entails integrating two distinct processes: (1) an exterior interaction process between the learners and their social, cultural or physical environment and (2) an interior mental element of development and assimilation (Illeris, 2018). If the meanings we captured in our research are shared, we will be encouraged to say that what emerged in our previous studies is also sharable within the scientific community.

The study reported in this chapter extracted an exploratory analysis of the major themes from the ethnography, interprofessional practice and SNA literature. A bibliometric software package, VOSviewer, was used to search for significant co-citations and keywords such as 'ethnography', 'hospitals', 'interprofessional' and 'social network analysis' as extracted from the web of knowledge on Microsoft Research API (https://msr-apis.portal.azure-api.net/). VOSviewer 1.4.0. is a software package developed by the University of Leiden. It creates distance-based bibliometric maps as diagrams, where the space between two keywords signals the intensity of their relationship (van Eck and Waltman, 2014).

The questions VOSviewer helped address are: (1) Within a given scientific subject, what are the key topics or study fields? (2) What is the relationship between these topics or fields? (Waltman et al., 2010). This process is called bibliographic network analysis (Waltman, van Eck and Noyons, 2010). During the construction of a bibliographic network, the nodes representing a single concept or word in a bibliometric network in the distance-based approach are placed so that the space between two nodes or ideas or words approximates their relatedness (van Eck and Waltman, 2010, 2017). A shorter length indicates a stronger relationship, although, in many circumstances, elements on distance-based maps are distributed unevenly (van Eck and Waltman, 2010, 2017). The closer the two nodes are, the more related they are (van Eck and Waltman, 2010, 2017). The NVIVO software analysis extracted the generalisations (QSR International Pty Ltd., 2020) from the summative narrative obtained by merging the targeted words extracted by VOSviewer (Figure 6.1).

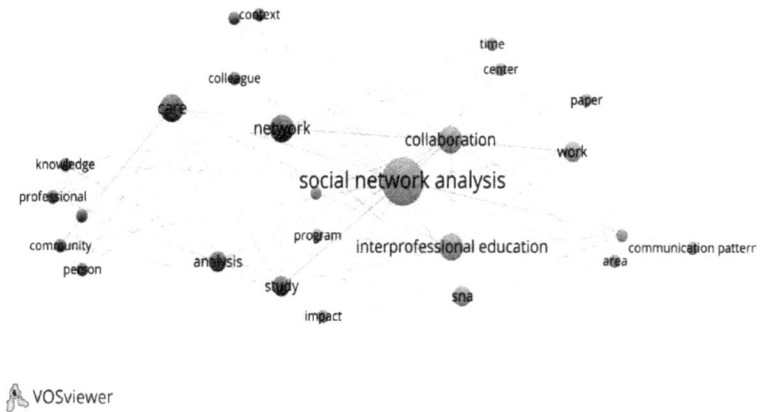

Figure 6.1. – VOSviewer extracts co-occurring words and concepts from selected keywords in the world of knowledge shown in a network. In the figure, the keywords are 'social network analysis' and 'interprofessional'. Each colour represents a cluster of meanings. The size of a bullet is proportional to the frequency of citation of the word to which it pertains (Lazzari, McAleer and Rabottini, 2022).

Findings

In the study reported in this chapter, VOSviewer extracted 542 manuscripts from the primary keywords. This was followed by the NVIVO thematic analysis, which generated the prevailing clusters. When the themes linked to SNA in hospitals and healthcare were searched, the international bibliography related 'social network analysis' to 'evidence-based practice'. When the co-occurrence of the word 'interprofessional' was investigated, the web of knowledge found that the co-cited words were 'network', 'knowledge', 'collaboration', 'communication pattern' and 'reciprocity'. In the following step, we used NVIVO to create narratives from the clusters generated from the co-occurring words. The results confirmed that an ethnographic assessment of nursing teamwork and SNA could help capture knowledge-sharing patterns in interprofessional teams, summarise the centralisation of information and explore forms of knowledge-sharing. These factors promote EBP (Evidence

Based Practice) in nursing and integrated skills under a collaborative approach to patient care (Figures 6.2. and 6.3.).

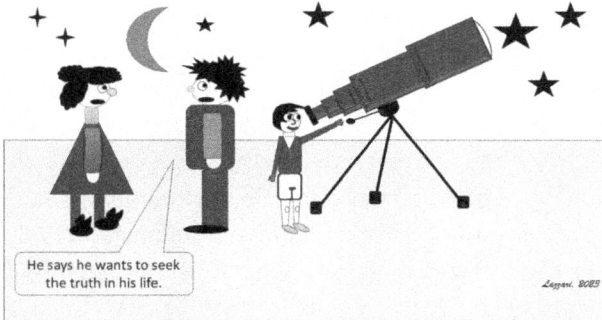

Figure 6.2. – Widely exploring the existing literature on a specific topic guides researchers' investigative vision.

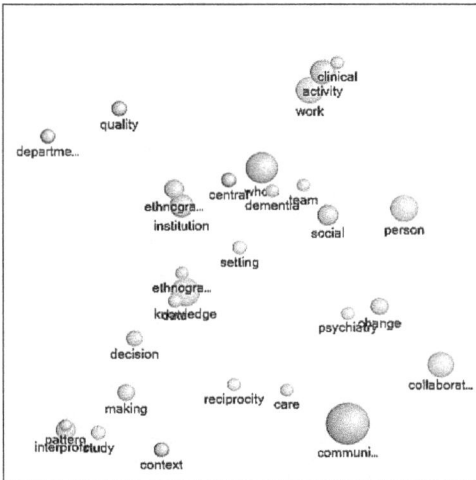

Figure 6.3. – NVIVO clustering of total words extracted by VOSviewer according to generalisations (Lazzari, McAleer and Rabottini, 2022)

Our study also confirmed the importance of SNA in capturing social networks and interprofessional care in healthcare. It also established the centrality of collaborative respect, reciprocity and shared knowledge in interprofessional practice in healthcare. Moreover, our analysis reinforced the status of *ethnographic observation* in portraying the target *behaviours* of interprofessional teams. More obtrusive attitude surveys might not reflect interpersonal relationship 'dynamics' but could instead extract staff's feelings. Furthermore, clinical governance in healthcare monitors outcomes and practices by measuring and analysing personnel's performances and acts using unobtrusive ethnographic observations. The goal is the patient's progress and care.

The results of the current study also confirm the influence of *communication* on HCP networks and the community. Also central is the concept of *unity,* the network's configuration regarding relationship patterns and the individuals' ideas, suggesting the need to focus on individuals (professionals or patients) in their totality. In addition, the study highlighted the concept of barriers. When these findings are matched with what is already known in the literature, it emerges that to promote integrated practice in health care and to create a combined achievement and practice-based evidence, practitioners should be mindful of communication barriers to interactions and collaborative efforts.

Middle-range theories

The MRTs that emerged from combining the current study's findings with our previous research outcomes are as follows.

MRT 1

Knowledge management and knowledge-sharing can guide HCPs in interprofessional teams regarding patient-focused EBP (Lazzari, Shoka, Papanna and Mousalidis, 2017). As our professional regulatory organisations advocate, there is an emerging recommendation that practice-based evidence achieved through interprofessional practice and scholarship can promote patients' personhood and lead to outcomes promoting evidence-based practice (Lazzari and Thomas, 2018).

MRT 2

Learning interprofessional practice can reinforce collaborative care in HCPs. Ethnographic research is the most productive approach to assessing target behaviours in coordinated care (Lazzari, 2018).

MRT 3

Promoting reciprocity, information and knowledge-sharing in interprofessional teams and focusing on the work context or settings of the service user and service providers help boost patient safety, health and interprofessional practice; these are also the goals of clinical governance and quality improvement in healthcare organisations (Lazzari and Rabottini, 2021). Furthermore, interprofessional teams in organisations constantly change their assets and set-up, which makes team members feel satisfied if changes correspond to their expectations or unhappy if new interpersonal relationships are detrimental to them (Figure 6.4.).

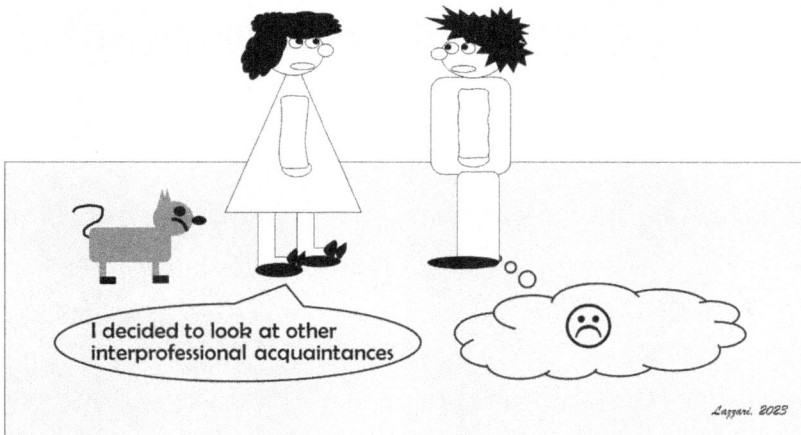

Figure 6.4 – In healthcare organisations, interprofessional relationships are vibrant and constantly changing.

Our reflections *on* action, professional growth and a way to change

One of the findings extracted from our analysis is that the web of science (WOS) links the concept of 'interprofessional' to the ideas of 'collaboration', 'network', 'reciprocity', 'knowledge', 'centre' and 'care' (Lazzari, McAleer and Rabottini, 2022). The WOS confirmed our MRTs and ideas about the link between interprofessional practice and patient care; in functional interprofessional groups, there is reciprocity in sharing knowledge and democratic collaboration among team members

(Lazzari, McAleer and Rabottini, 2022). We suggest that policymakers reinforce interprofessional practice and collaboration by facilitating the circulation of vital information and knowledge about patients within interprofessional teams. The outcome is improved quality of care and enhanced patient safety (NHS England, 2014). In the next chapter, we will explore how to promote clinical handovers in interprofessional teams.

CHAPTER 7

Interprofessional Handover

Abstract

The current chapter explores a critical side of interprofessional relationships. Clinical handovers allow team members to share vital information in the care of communal patients. Understanding the power and complexities of providing complete handovers is the basis of professionalism in healthcare settings. The chapter analyses the study, Lazzari, C. (2023) 'Theoretical Frameworks of Clinical Handovers in Healthcare Settings', *Research Highlights in Disease and Health Research* Vol. 4, pp.125–147.

Our reflection *in* action

The following passage is a quote from our chronicle, which we kept when we conducted this study and worked in interprofessional teams. The excerpt encapsulates the issue that prompted our research question and the writing of this chapter. It is an ad verbatim extraction of our conversation with colleagues in healthcare settings.

> «Although we might adopt all strategies for proficient interprofessional care, some primary data about patient care is missing. We discovered that some handovers were crafted according to our framework and professional experiences. Instead, others were piecemeal and lacked significant aspects to allow us to understand what was

happening to patients. Our teams have sufficient expertise to produce the basic information (written or electronic) necessary to transfer the patient's data within the unit. We need more clarity about what is expected when communicating clinical data in our interprofessional teams».

Introduction

Having reliable clinical handovers helps reduce threats to population health. In this case, coordination between teams of HCPs through a shared handover framework helps diffuse knowledge and data to understand multifaceted medical conditions in shared customers and populations. However, one of the major contributors to adverse clinical outcomes is a communication breakdown in interprofessional teams, especially when there is an interprofessional handover. Instead, the introduction, situation, background, assessment, and recommendation (ISBAR or simply SBAR) communication tool was created to improve handover efficiency and is commonly believed to improve patient safety and quality of care (Lazzari, 2023).

Table 7.1. Reflection in action in teamwork and strategies.

The actual event	Considering it when it was occurring	Settings where applied	Acting without delay (motto)	Choosing how to respond at the moment
The healthcare team does not equally craft the handover to its standards.	We find that some information is missing to conduct a proper patient assessment.	MDT meetings and electronic patient records.	Adhering to a standard handover helps you help others.	Make team members adopt the ISBAR framework. Do the same yourself.
Different healthcare teams appear to adopt diversified handover frameworks.	Working in liaison teams and having to communicate with colleagues from other specialty areas	General hospitals.	Handover frameworks are all the same, although their content changes.	Craft your handover according to the ISBAR and make information simple, straightforward, legible, and meaningful for those who read it.

It is also reported that communication bottlenecks occur when health professionals communicate more prevalently with co-workers from the same educational or professional background. In this case, information and knowledge about communal patients might not circulate consistently within interprofessional teams (Lazzari, 2023).

Clinical handovers (CHs) represent the act of transferring (verbal, written or electronic) information and liability about patients between health carers (WHO, 2007). A *handover* involves moving responsibility from the sender to the receiver via interaction and interventions to reduce ambiguity about a patient's condition (Kim and Seomun, 2020). Through CHs, HCPs aim to clarify anything related to patient care management and assessment in a specific context and setting (Kim and Seomun, 2020). Therefore, during handovers, information about a patient is shared through communication among caregivers, within a team of carers, and between the hospital and the patient's family or the patient himself (WHO, 2007). Hence, information about a patient is shared during *handover communication* with another caregiver, a new team of carers, the patient, and the patient's family (WHO, 2007).

Handovers epitomise oral, written or electronic notes about a patient's current clinical conditions, treatment plans, and any assessment and clinical outcomes generated by the professional developing the handovers (WHO, 2007). Furthermore, *nursing handover* occurs when one nurse transfers to another nurse (via oral or electronic communication) the responsibility for the care and any information about a patient, usually after a shift–typically making three handovers per day (Smeulers, Lucas and Vermeulen, 2014). In more detail, a *clinical handover* (1) is the communication of data about patients; (2) it allows a continuity of care within the team, the transfer of responsibility for assessment and treatment, the sharing of any information about clinical conditions and reviews about a patient allowing the continuity of care; and (3) a CH also consents shared care plans, and transfer of the responsibilities for assessment and care to another member of the team or other teams to whom the handover is directed or who have equal responsibility towards the patient (Government of Western Australia Department of Health, 2022; Rickard et al., 2022).

Therefore, a CH ('clinical hand-off' in America) refers to the temporary (e.g., daily clinical notes, patient progress, liaison assessment) or final (e.g., discharge from hospital, referral to another team or structure) of partial or total information and responsibility for care to another member of the professional team or a group from another setting, hospital or community (Australian Medical Association, 2022). During routine daily practice, CH is conducted in various fashions: (1) during verbal handovers, healthcare professionals talk with each other about a patient; (2) sometimes, nurses talk about a patient while reading relative notes about a patient presentation, assessment or clinical conditions; (3) in some cases, handovers are conducted at the patient's bedside so that patient presentation, symptoms and conditions can help complete the required information (Australian Medical Association, 2022).

Clinical data about patients represent the central information that is communicated during handovers. Information is any data transmitted or conveyed between persons by a mutual system of representations, symbols or behaviours (Merriam-Webster Dictionary Online, 2023). Broken communication links in verbal and written handovers about patients and between healthcare providers are responsible for 25% to 40% of adverse patient care events, 27% of cases of medical misconduct and over 70% of warning clinical incidents (Eggins and Slade, 2015). An investigation of 23,000 medical malpractice lawsuits found that more than 7,000 were attributed to communication failures among caregivers during patient handovers, resulting in about 2,000 preventable casualties and 80% of serious medical errors (The Joint Commission, 2023). In research on 16,165 electronic data in Michigan, among the significant drawbacks in interprofessional communication were missing necessary data, overlooked communication goals, skewed physical or temporal situations or contexts of the message, omitted key participants and unclear or lost information (Umberfield et al., 2019).

Face-to-face interprofessional communication, a meeting, ward round, hand-off, or spontaneous discussion are synchronous CHs (Conn et al., 2009). Asynchronous communications occur on whiteboards, in written progress reports, in electronic patients' notes or via the ordering of medications (Conn et al., 2009). The SBAR (situation, background, assessment and recommendation) and its derivate ISBAR (SBAR +

introduction) and K-SBAR (SBAR + Kindness) frameworks are based on the four or five stages of patients' handover (Breen et al., 2019; Burgess et al., 2020; Institute for Healthcare Improvement, 2023; Müller et al., 2018):

- *introduction:* the person who writes the handover provides information about the own identity and role and why s/he is providing the data; it also introduces the information about the patient, inclusive of name, age, gender and current location;
- *situation*: the expert presents the patient's history and summarises any ongoing issues, progress and any relevant information the team must know about, for example, what brought the patient to the hospital;
- *background*: the expert provides relevant background information on the patient's present illness and critical incidents contributing to the current problem, including past physical and mental illnesses;
- *assessment*: is the core of the evaluation and clinical analysis where the professionals express their point of view on the problem(s), give their professional impression of what they believe is occurring to the patient and suggest a possible solution(s);
- *recommendation*: the professional offers a proposed line of action to address the problem in analysis and improve the presentation (Figure 7.1.).

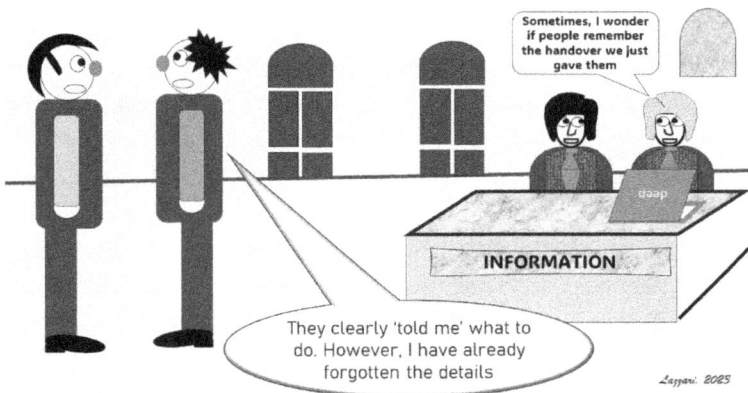

Figure 7.1. – There is a high probability that verbal handovers might be misinterpreted or forgotten.

A constructionist approach to handovers

The social construction of handovers and the sharing of patient information undergoes several stages where the target of attention are 'patients', 'service users', 'families' and others. The social construction of meanings about patients is regulated by the professional background of those who generate verbal, written or electronic notes about them. Especially in medical or psychiatric settings, the patient presentation characterises the object of knowledge sharing. Therefore, information about a patient becomes a social construction in which a clinical (re) production is shared during handover communication and interprofessional meetings (Mathisen et al., 2016). Handovers can thus be seen as essential to teams' existence and corporate goals as they distribute participation positions by constructing the meaning and needs of organisational users (e.g., patients) (Mathisen et al., 2016).

However, sometimes, CHs have missing information in some or most parts. Therefore, from one side, the professional obligation is to use the best of one's knowledge to provide a complete CH. Conversely, practitioners might adapt to the local (unspoken) rules of handling patient information but generate clinical notes with little impact on knowledge sharing and adding minimal meaning to patients' clinical assessments and recommendations.

When we hand over as healthcare professionals and teachers to our high-ranking and junior colleagues, we adhere to and complete what we feel are the demands of the situation. Yet, completeness in the communication exchange requires checking that the message was delivered, understood, and somewhat acknowledged by the recipient/s of the handovers. For instance, an email without ensuring that the intended message was understood and acted on is not a handover.

Yet, several health carers might have different clinical backgrounds, collaborate from various organisations, and thus abide by norms that might not bridge their interacting teams. Hence, although the standardisation of CHs has occurred through training and geographical/ organisational location, gaps might still exist (Lazzari, 2023). For example, team members construct their social reality according to how CHs should be created (Lazzari, 2023). This process of individual and unstandardised interpretations of CHs leaves room for multiple variations of the expected norm to conform to generate the final and agreed-upon handover (Lazzari, 2023).

Middle-range theories

The current chapter proposes several MRTs in CH.

MRT 1

In the group of interacting and communicating health carers, the individual intentionality disappears when using handover communication to share essential data (verbal or electronic) about patients (Lazzari, 2023). Standardised regulations on CHs instead attract uniqueness in CH. Furthermore, there are standard operating procedures (SOP) about patient information disclosure and collective participation (Lazzari, 2023). SOP also regulate any professional socialising instrument (handover) to communicate; this process falls into the organisational and corporate guidelines of how to share information in good practice and interprofessional healthcare (Lazzari, 2023).

MRT 2

Gatekeepers and high-ranking HCPs might have a preferential and pivotal role in interprofessional communication. However, not all information management can and should be the prerogative of a limited number of professionals. Instead, for social osmosis, every piece of information pertinent to a team should be diffused so that the final distribution is even and does not impact the team's clinical and professional goals. On the contrary, data centralisation risks are team imbalance, silos management, and organisational entropy (Lazzari, 2004).

MRT 3

Members of an interprofessional team aiming for a specific goal need to communicate by adhering to the same and shared meanings, symbolic language, jargon expressions, and professional terms. For example, the same technical word can assume different meanings according to the characteristics of the team where the word circulates. On the contrary, by adapting to the exact symbolic representations, people in interprofessional teams undergo a progressive economy of language in expressing and sharing concepts and reduce the time required for a piece of information to be deciphered correctly. Nonetheless, due to the formation of interpersonal hubs, accessing private and professional jargon might need some form of social trust, induction or initiation, which is not immediately available to all newcomers in a group (Figure 7.2.).

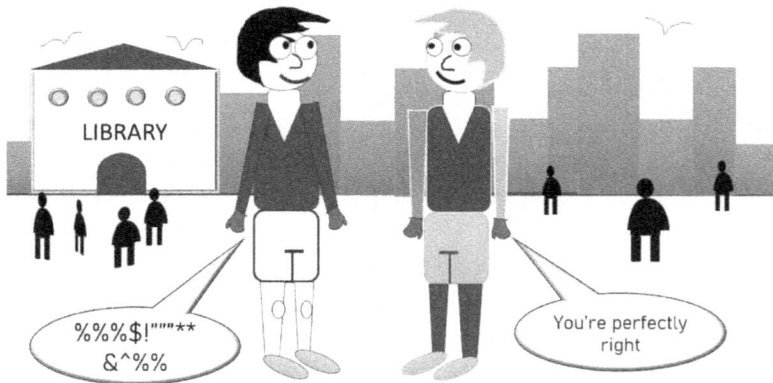

Lazzari, 2023

Figure 7.2. – There is a high probability that sharing symbolic, value, social and professional background helps decipher interprofessional speech that outsiders might find unclear.

Our reflections *on* action, professional growth and a way to change

Communicating patients' data properly to colleagues and providing complete clinical handovers is an act of professionalism and reduces health inequalities and the likelihood of medical errors. Furthermore, CHs advance teams' performance and reduce uncertainties in clinical practice. Hence, we endeavour to be understood in our interprofessional communication as we know that ISBAR applies in every setting, not solely clinical. Furthermore, through daily routine and checking, we can feel confident that we can deliver the proper data about any situation with an economy of our efforts and optimisation of message clarity to reach our intentions and corporate goals.

Conclusions

As seen in this chapter, clinical handovers represent the instrument of communication used by healthcare interprofessional teams to operate according to their goals and organisational requirements. As most of this communication is either verbal, non-verbal or paraverbal, gaining access to shared meanings and jargon is required to tackle higher levels of interprofessional communication and to collaborate toward the shared goals of a team. In addition, there is also a risk that people who are acquainted use the same private language whose meaning is unclear to those who do not belong to the group or specialist team (e.g., a medical team and a team in psychiatry). If this event happens in highly functional interprofessional teams aiming at patient care and safety, an impasse in communication and data sharing might occur. Therefore, healthcare organisations must strive to provide HCPs with a common language of communication specific to each specialist team working in primary and secondary care. Furthermore, newcomers in a team need to have a period of induction to learn how the team communicates.

CHAPTER 8

Conclusions

Aim

During our career development, our path was not always straight. Each day, we had to surmount constant perils or face exciting challenges in interprofessional teamwork. We believe that each person working in multidisciplinary teams can promote change, create better working conditions and offer healthier patient care. As previously analysed, the intricate web of organisational relations found in interprofessional teams, with the different arrays of communication and information exchange, can be captured by conducting a network analysis of the interpersonal choices. In this chapter, we now explore how we implemented changes in our WBL based on the MRTs we crafted from the public works presented in this book.

This book has allowed us to make wider-ranging considerations by challenging ourselves with novel audiences, structures of concepts and ideas that the academy offers. Whereas it has underpinned sufficiently theory to practice, this newly acquired knowledge has also questioned the nature of interprofessional education's and practice's status quo, possibly in a novel way.

The practitioner-researcher approach

In Clarke's *scientist-practitioner model*, a social scientist proceeds from describing an individual instance of the research goal (e.g., problems, people, events) to explain the phenomena under study and then to the final intervention in the social scenario (cited by Miller and Frederickson, 2006). In Shapiro's *scientist-practitioner model*, experts embrace their profession's scientific foundation to base their therapeutic approaches on evidence while considering their research's applicability and translational value (Maree, 2020; Shapiro, 2002). By working in a scientist-practitioner role, we applied critical thinking to our practice, employed proven treatments, assessed programmes and procedures, and used methodologies and techniques supported by our research (Jones and Mehr, 2007). As scientist-practitioners, we seamlessly blended the science of and theories in social domains into our practice to help teams and patients (Jones and Mehr, 2007). The result is the dynamic interplay between *practice-based evidence (PBE)* and *evidence-based practice (EBP)*.

Work-based learning in our academic pathway

Our work-based learning has helped us integrate theory with an applicative flavour, empowering reflections about our findings that could be valued for healthcare teams, service users and any other setting where persons work as a team to reach common goals. We did not split our time between our daily work and learning. The two processes progressed jointly and enhanced each other to achieve EBP linked to PBE.

WBL refers to the knowledge acquired in the workplace or from tackling problems (Lester and Costley, 2010). Most of this learning is not certified or publicly acknowledged, though much of it may be; it entails learning while doing one's job to further one's professional goals and interests, as a result of workplace coaching or training or as a means of problem-solving (Lester and Costley, 2010). It overlaps with experiential, continuing professional development (CPD) and informal or nonformal learning (Lester and Costley, 2010). WBL occurs in various ways, including unstructured, ad hoc, retroactively and serendipitously; it may also be organised and prepared in advance by the student, the organisation, a school, a business or a trade union (Lester and Costley, 2010). The importance of WBL and face-to-face learning is reported in another study, where this approach helped clinical support workers in psychiatric settings expand practice skills and reflective learning abilities (Kemp et al., 2016).

WBL and associated reflective practice helped us develop our problem-solving skills, our skills in formulating MRTs, our aptitude for using a narrative to dialogue with healthcare organisations and our aspiration to share our findings with our colleagues and the scientific community. Moreover, WBL enhanced our understanding of how to change what we perceived could be problematic conditions for effective collaborative care. Argyris and Schön (1974) claimed that people who act intentionally—that is, people who know what to do when faced with a given situation to achieve an intended result—use theories of action or 'theory-in-use'. Such people know the nature of the result they need to attain, the appropriate action that must be taken to achieve it and the assumptions contained in the theory of action (Argyris and Schön, 1974).

In our research on interprofessional practice, we focused on the actions of social persons to understand the theory-in-use concerning interprofessional relationships. Since the pictorial representation of behaviours can represent social networks' dynamics, the theories behind these nets could be inferred from the configuration of interpersonal links. There was no need to extract motivations and beliefs to understand and classify interprofessional behaviours in organisations. The more we studied, the more interprofessional theories we could draw upon. The concept of continuity in WBL states that the impact of an event is cumulative since it is formed by previous experiences, which in turn influence subsequent ones (Schmidt, 2010). It was, thus, central for us to be immersed in *settings and cultures similar* to the ones we extracted from our subsequent research. We were members of the teams that mirrored those reported in our studies. Dewey introduced the concept of *interaction*, suggesting that individuals create opinions from experience when interacting with their physical and social environments (Schmidt, 2010). Our wealth of experience in the field helped us complete the current book.

Our studies reported in the current manuscript have deepened our understanding of daily practice in interprofessional teams. With encouragement from our colleagues, we used our knowledge and intuition to create viable and applicative hypotheses about interprofessional practice. While completing the current book, we matured to a probably higher level of learning by focusing on our published work. Moreover, we acquired valuable experience to develop possibly convincing and practical theories on our areas of interest, such as interprofessional teamwork in healthcare settings. Our research could thus be conceptualised and executed intellectually, rigorously and robustly through the publications linked to the current book and its chapters (Costley and Lester, 2011).

Therefore, as we progressed in our study, the experience grew more captivating and our thinking more divergent as we could perceive how a discursive and inductive explanation of our research could open new avenues for understanding social phenomena from a broader perspective. We felt that we could cross the regional boundaries of our clinical settings and use our analysis to attempt a scientific dialogue that could be understood from different theoretical and professional viewpoints.

One PhD candidate in professional doctorates stated that the practitioner-researcher goal of a study is to promote change in a specific setting of practice, where the unique and explicit motivations of people might make a difference (Costley and Armsby, 2007a). We have always been compelled by social phenomena and the related events that link people and their surrounding environments. Our choice of people-based professions (medicine, academy, teaching) reflects this. Moreover, as mentioned before, we developed a particular interest in studying social networks because of our professional background working within academia and for clinical and healthcare teams. Our values are also social: we like to think pluralistically, be treated democratically, and be valued as members of interprofessional and interdisciplinary groups.

Natural selection has instilled in us a set of innate proclivities that drive us to be social, cooperative and altruistic; these orientations also serve as the yardstick by which we judge the actions of others (Decety and Steinbeis, 2020). We wanted to advocate a scientific-practitioner approach, learn to think judiciously, use the information to influence our activities and utilise clinical practice to inform our inquiry (Kison, Moorer and Villarosa, 2015). Our context shaped the direction of our learning and different forms of reflection, such as re-analysing our long-held assumptions (see Taylor and Hamdy, 2013). Our constant pedagogical tact of personal understanding to be redistributed as social learning suggests that scholarship can occur because of educational activities, such as clarifying occurring events, solving questions and reflective knowledge development (see Fiorella and Mayer, 2013). In these instances, the culture promoters, perhaps ourselves, critically reflect on their understanding of the material object of education (see Fiorella and Mayer, 2013).

Generalisability and transferability

The current book, in its structure, uses somewhat an interpretivist approach also by applying Guba and Lincoln's (1986) criteria of (1) *credibility* that we reached by prolonged engagement, persistent observations, and triangulation of methods, (2) *transferability* by employing a thick description of events, (3) *dependability* and *confirmability* by applying methodological triangulation. Here, they are described in more detail. Our applied *axiology* was to raise awareness and develop democratic participation in interprofessional practices; our *ontology* is relativism, which acknowledges multiple and subjective interpretations of social realities of persons who dynamically interacted in their daily routine; the settings and definitions were thus contextual; our *epistemology* and methods for the research that compiled the book were interactive with us as researchers and participant-observers of the social interactions reported; our *methodology* as applied to the manuscript *on its own* is somewhat interpretive with logical and well-described contexts (see Collis & Hussey, 2014). Moreover, the descriptive narrative that sustained the explanation of the studies reported in the book is similar to an exploratory enquiry. Our documented research to which the manuscript refers was based on a naturalistic, unobtrusive ethnographic approach. We, as researchers, were participant observers and sometimes applied Goffman's unsystematic observation protocol (Goffman, 1963a) during the initial stages of our observations. Goffman's frame analysis is centred on understanding micro-society behaviours and studying local social interactions (Persson, 2018). The steps were necessary to achieve the generalisability and transferability of our findings.

Generalisability (G) of the current findings (and the studies reported in the book) represents the extension and conclusions from our studies conducted on a sample group of mental health practitioners to the general population of HCPs. Our quantitative research (in mixed-method studies) offered the best foundation for G. Generalisability has the following characteristics, (1) G is based on probability values, our research findings were accepted if the statistical significance was more significant than the value *alpha* (statistical power) set at probability equal 0.05, meaning that a researcher makes less than 5% chance of committing an error in generalising the results from the research sample to the general population, (2) G was crucial to produce evidence-based practice by extending the results to populations, settings, interventions and periods other than those under study, (3) G was also based on *ecological validity* which measured how closely research results reflected conditions in the real world, (4) G hit its target when the *sample*–the group of persons who participated in a study from the target population– was sufficiently representative of the *population*–the collection of individuals (health carers) who all share a crucial attribute–in general, and (5) if research findings were statistically significant, they could be generalisable from the sample to the (new) population and settings maintaining its effectiveness (Barnes et al., 2005; Wang, Moss and Hiller, 2006; Polit and Beck, 2010; Burchett, Umoquit and Dobrow, 2011; Kamper, 2020; APA Dictionary Online, 2023; Figure 8.1).

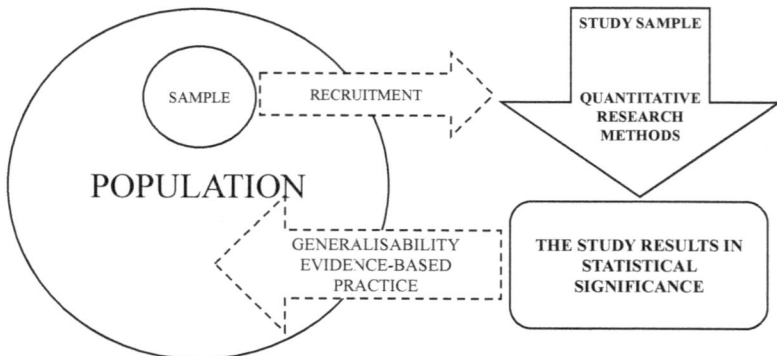

Figure 8.1. – The link between population and generalisation (Adapted from Kamper 2020, p. 45)

To allow the transferability of our research findings, we also endeavoured to provide a *thick description* of events and settings using the best evidence from mixed-method studies, WBL experiences and matured PBE. Albert Einstein mentioned that not all things that can be numbered matter, and not all things that matter can be measured (Anonym., 2023).

Transferability refers to the accomplishment of a researcher/reader comparing and applying the research findings from one circumstance in another analogous setting he is familiar with (Barnes et al., 2005; Wang, Moss and Hiller, 2006). The researcher, having much knowledge as possible of the original studies, deduces that the initial research results are comparable and *applicable*–the probability that an intervention could be applied in novel and explicit settings–to his circumstances as there are significant similarities between the two scenarios and interventions (Barnes et al., 2005; Wang, Moss and Hiller, 2006). The researcher/reader also assumes that there is a high probability that the original study's discoveries can be reproduced in new and particular settings, maintaining their effectiveness; Furthermore, qualitative research methods like ethnography and case studies are crucial for transferability (Barnes et al., 2005; Wang, Moss and Hiller, 2006; Figure 8.2, Table 8.1).

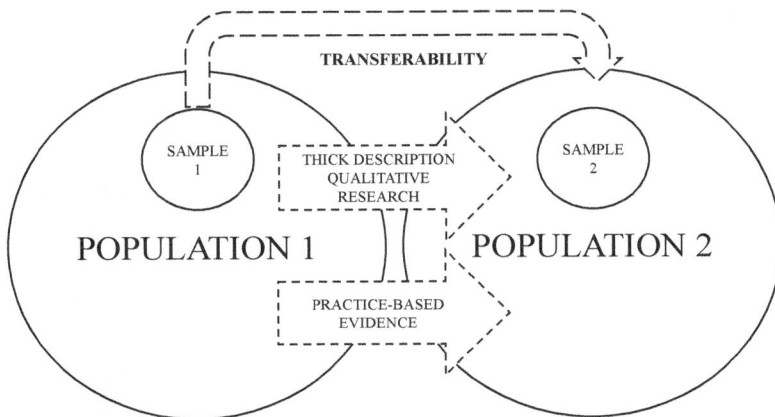

Figure 8.2. – The link between sample and transferability, as used in the book.

Table 8.1.– Generalisable and transferable results from the book chapters and our model.

Public Works	Research Method	Generalisable	Transferable
Chapter 1 – Introduction	Theoretical basis of the current book		X
Study Chapter 2	Descriptive and qualitative thick analysis; theoretical paper		X
Study Chapter 3	Mixed Method of Social Network Analysis and Ethnographic Confirmation	X	X
Study Chapter 4	Mixed Method of Social Network Analysis and Ethnographic Confirmation	X	X
Study Chapter 5	Quantitative Method	X	X
Study Chapter 6	Qualitative Bibliometric Analysis		X
Study Chapter 7	Qualitative analysis and theoretical exploration		X
Chapter 8 – Conclusions	Theoretical aspects of WBL, EVP and PBE		X

The question that transferability answers is about how successfully the research's findings educate healthcare contexts that vary from those in which the primary study was completed (Kitto, Chesters and Garbich, 2008). The studies reported in the current book were mainly based on our mixed-method and qualitative research to allow generalisability and transferability. Therefore, the present manuscript and our aim by using transferability and generalisability was to draw conclusions that may apply to comparable circumstances, settings, teams and geographical locations (Burchett, Umoquit and Dobrow, 2011; Nikolopoulou, 2013). These processes lead to our Practice-Based Evidence.

We used **Practice-Based Evidence** (PBE) as practitioner-researchers to make our arguments convincing to a broader audience and conduct ground-breaking research to enhance and implement (interprofessional) practice by recognising the importance of context and situatedness (Costley and Fulton, 2015). Transferability and thick descriptions helped endorse our PBE as described in the current book by producing, (1) research closer and tailored to actual circumstances of practice and reaching high external validity by including all participants with a particular feature while analysing treatments associated with better outcomes for specific target populations, (2) recognising that people are multifaceted and do not fit the cause-and-effect model of science, (3) using prospective, observational and cohort studies, (4) allowing for many simultaneous treatments and target population characteristics that corresponded to actual clinical practice, (5) using information from natural environments to characterise the timing and substance of treatments that are linked to improved results (including patient-reported outcomes) for participants with specific characteristics, (6) applying *how-to* questions about implementation of interventions and strategies and *what* questions about barriers or keys to success in using interventions and approaches, (7) employing subliminal processes of reassessment and adjustment involving backward reference to books, research articles and other trusted sources of knowledge, and (8) enhancing evidence in areas in which trial designs are not appropriate (Green, 2008; Gabbay and Le May, 2010; Swisher, 2010; Horn and Gassaway, 2010; Leeman and Sandelowski, 2012; Holmqvist, Philips and Barkham, 2015; Figure 8.3).

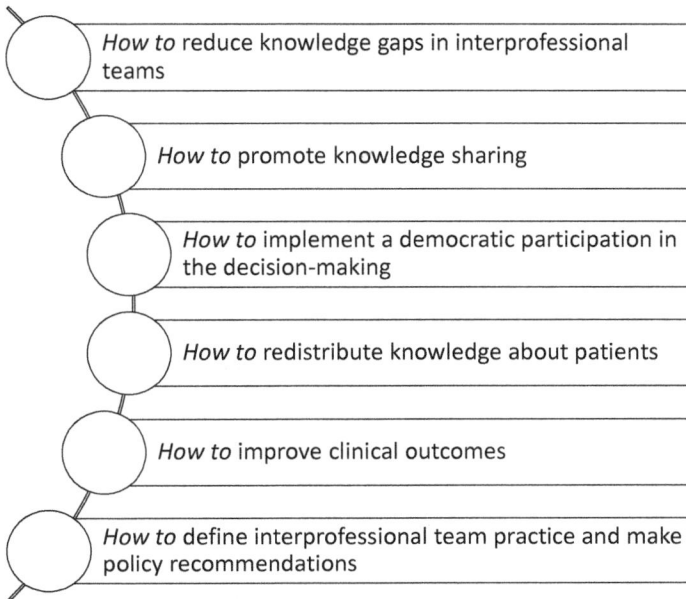

How to reduce knowledge gaps in interprofessional teams

How to promote knowledge sharing

How to implement a democratic participation in the decision-making

How to redistribute knowledge about patients

How to improve clinical outcomes

How to define interprofessional team practice and make policy recommendations

Figure 8.3. – Key foci in PBE in interprofessional practice.

We used **thick descriptions**[1] of micro-societies to define and explain how observed behaviours within their specific context occurred (APA, 2023; Ponterotto, 2006). Through a thick analysis, observed behaviours become understandable to outsiders; the aim is to relate theoretically and analytically general and abstract patterns and qualities of community life in society (APA, 2023; Ponterotto, 2006). We adopted the PIO (Population, Intervention, Outcomes) framework to ease our thick descriptions and help us endorse PBE and its transferability:

- *service users*: elderly persons in psychogeriatrics units, working age population in general adult psychiatry, children and adolescents in psychiatric hospitals, patients with HIV/AIDS in infectious diseases departments, customers of prominent corporations, and street children in slums of developing countries;
- *service providers in interprofessional teams*: mental health teams, clinical units in infectious diseases wards, HCPs, employees of large corporations, and volunteers in non-governmental organisations;
- *our role* when observations occurred, we were in healthcare or university professions;
- *interventions or teamwork behaviours*: interprofessional clinical practice, interprofessional education, corporate interactions, volunteer teams;
- *outcomes* were patient care and safety, interventions in rural and suburban areas in developing countries, counselling of terminal patients, support of homeless people, and intervention and education programs for children in developing countries.

Therefore, due to the collective nature of our team knowledge, our PBE was strictly linked to WBL. Knowledge creation in WBL was influenced by "real-world" and "real-time" requirements, and it took place in diverse and opposing settings where it was often shared, co-produced, and co-developed via professional practice (Costley and

---

1 A thick description captures the non-observable contextual understandings that give meaning to an action or social event (Reference: Kostova, I. (2017) 'Definition of Thick Description', The Wiley-Blackwell Encyclopedia of Social Theory, pp. 1–2. Available at: https://doi.org/10.1002/9781118430873.est077 (Accessed: 24 August 2023).

Dikerdem, 2011). We acquired this knowledge through autoethnography, which was to *enter the world and go native, whereby* we lived with those being studied (see Hayes and Fulton, 2015). As auto-ethnographers, we wrote about our culture, the culture of our place of employment, and our daily lives (see Hayes and Fulton, 2015). As Anderson (2006) advised, we, as researchers, are part of the investigation area and engaged with the informants (see Hayes and Fulton, 2015). Our objective was to acquire *tacit* knowledge or expertise that the teams and we obtained implicitly or unconsciously inside our organisations; this knowledge entailed competency that was not officially acknowledged but necessary for our organisation to operate (see Chisholm and Holifield, 2003). To increase an organisation's future knowledge capital, it is crucial to capture the information achieved by tacit knowledge and transform it into explicit knowledge (Holifield, Clarke and Jones, 2011). It is argued that successful learning and developing personal/professional competence are intimately tied to the transfer of tacit information and tacit knowledge in organisations (Holifield, Chisholm and Harris, 2008).

Evidence-Based Practice (EBP) intended by the current book demanded that decisions regarding clinical treatments be backed by the best, existing, practical, promptly accessible and applicable evidence; these choices were taken by individuals like us who were involved in the interventions or treatments supported by the implied and overt knowledge of those providing care and considering the available assets (Dawes et al., 2003). Consequently, the quantitative experimental (e.g., mixed-method) techniques reported in the studies scrutinised in each chapter were *also* used –after an initial stage of ethnographic/autoethnographic study– to test generated hypotheses (Carminati, 2018). We aimed to draw generalisable findings by now assuming the participation of an unbiased and objective researcher to reduce any potential forms of influence in the study (Carminati, 2018).

The traditional basis of EBP for quantitative studies uses a grading system positioning at the base (a lower degree of evidence) case series or reports, case-control studies, to then progress to cohort studies, randomised controlled studies and systematic review and meta-analysis at the top (Hassan et al., 2016). Similarly, the grading of qualitative research evidence starts from low-degree evidence in studies with one informant to a group study with rigorous methods (Tomlin and Borgetto, 2011). The studies reported in the chapters and related publications discussed in the book included case-control studies, cohort studies, exploratory and explanatory research, and rigorous group studies, positioning the result and text's findings from moderate to high degrees of EBP and PBE.

We have integrated the advice of The American Speech-Language-Hearing Association (2023) into EBP recommendations by merging three aspects, (1) clinical knowhow/skilled judgement that was the information, decision, and informed thinking gained through our preparation and qualified knowledge, (2) by employing the best evidence gleaned from scientific works (external evidence) and statistics and reflections collected in our setting (internal evidence), and (3) patient's or caregiver's standpoint as the specific collection of individual and social situations, ideals, requirements, and hopes. Therefore, there was a dynamic process of applying PBE to generate EBP and *vice versa* and confronting the outcomes with previous PBE for confirmation and improvement. The steps used to achieve EBP were (1) identifying our clinical inquiry, (2) gathering data, (3) evaluating the information, and (4) crafting our clinical decisions (practice) (American Speech-Language-Hearing Association, 2023). In a dynamic process, PBE informed EBP and backward, EBP improved the instruments for a deeper PBE. In the last stage, we thus employed the reverse steps (EBP to PBE) to advise our PBE by (1) re-reflecting on interprofessional decisions, practice and outcomes, (2) re-evaluating if there was evidence for the adopted interprofessional practice or if amendments were needed in observations and applications, (3) re-gathering the present evidence, and (4) reframing an applicative research question (Figure 8.4).

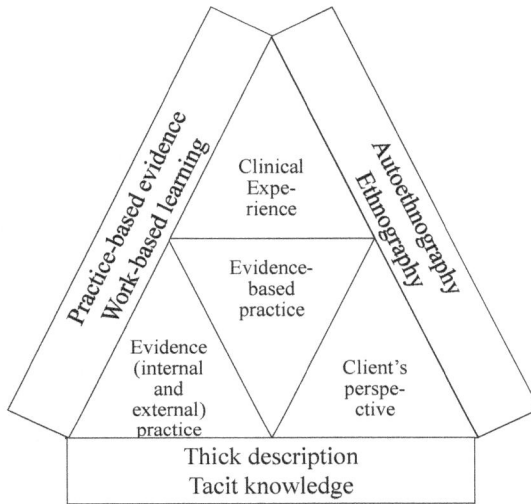

Figure 8.4. – The correlation between EBP and PBE as developed in the book (Figure adapted and modified from Bartgis and Bigfoot, 2010).

Autoplastic change

In interprofessional practice, each practitioner in a team works for the healthcare system. The leadership responsible for functional changes in interprofessional practice involved our direct and indirect collaborators and us in long-lasting growth (see Nikolou-Walker and Curley, 2012), resulting in improved care and a better work climate. In this sense, the constant reflective practice of WBL helped change us in the first instance. The insights we gained from research and observations broadened our understanding of our collaborative work with other team members. Thus, there has also been a dynamic change process from within in addition to changes in settings.

Changes that occur on the inside of a person, called *autoplastic* changes, are distinguished from those that appear on the outside, called *alloplastic* changes (Nicholls, 1984; Wainrib, 2005). To cope with stress, according to Ferenczi, one may either (1) try to modify one's external environment (alloplastic adaptation) or (2) try to change one's interior environment (autoplastic adaptation) (Ferenczi, 1994). When we started to operate autoplastically, we became operative, working with our skills to manage our integration in interprofessional teams. We tried to change from within through self-reflection and adapting to the complex social realities we were in contact with through an operative and self-determined strategy (see Merriam-Webster Dictionary, 2000a). Then, we moved to an alloplastic transformation and conducted proactive actions in our environment, aiming to understand the social networks in healthcare settings to establish a foundation to propose viable changes (see Merriam-Webster Dictionary, 2000b).

We represent our stages of change as follows: (1) first, there was our significant interest in changing the social networks we operated in, which generated (2) a sort of emotional tension that resulted in a better understanding of interpersonal dynamics, which led to (3) the first stage of personal adaptation, autoplastic, which improved our interpersonal skills and then resulted in (4) WBL, which culminated in (5) a personal change in our team interactions based on our newly acquired interpersonal skills. The loop continues with higher levels of interpersonal and interprofessional needs (Figure 8.5.).

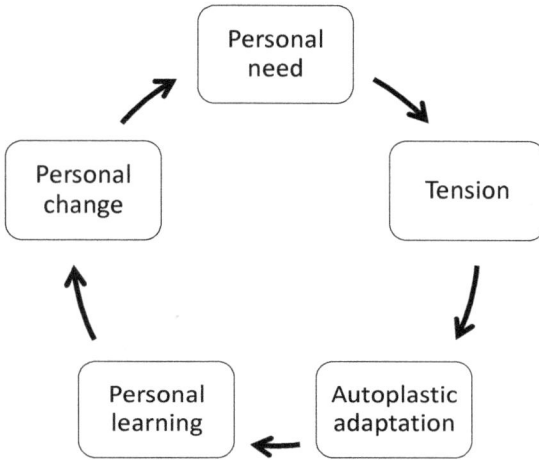

Figure 8.5.– Our theoretical model of autoplastic adaptation.

Alloplastic change

Living in social contexts with our own goals and where other people interact with each other to achieve shared aspirations, we were both observers and researchers. The loop of social change helped us think and act pluralistically. We identified ourselves with our teams, which made us perceive that we could address personal and professional needs only through pluralistic/group thinking. As long as a social condition was perceived, we also experienced social tension, a collective feeling that something needed to change in our interprofessional practices and skills. As we aimed to change pluralistically, we made some adaptations to our social environment, such as the regulations and job descriptions that guided our collaborative practice.

At this point, our learning became systemic. Each of us had the potential to become an active agent in an interprofessional network of people who mutually interacted with and influenced one another. In clinical teams, new social configurations were always desired, and those social arrangements that could help us become more effective in reaching organisational goals by supporting our feelings of job satisfaction were usually endorsed.

The more we could do professionally and the higher our roles and responsibilities in clinical and educational settings, the more we could be promoters of changes where we worked; this last was our alloplastic transformation. In a more literary way, alloplastic also means shaping or being shaped by external factors (such as the environment) (Merriam-Webster Dictionary, 2022a). Hence, a self-reflective practice coincides with autoplastic growth to deal successfully with the exterior (social) world (Merriam-Webster Dictionary, 2022a). These changes and insights culminated in the production of MRTs, as reported in this book. At this point, our teams had a poignant perception that we had engineered a systemic change, all working together with shared values and actions (Figure 8.6).

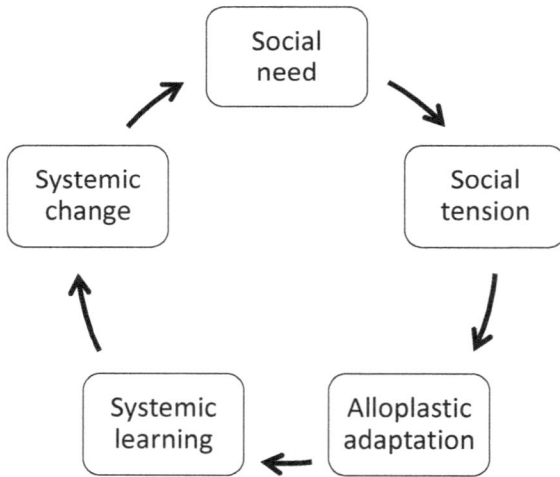

Figure 8.6. – A systemic model of alloplastic adaptation.

We also plan to disseminate the findings reported in this book. An unpublished study is a significant loss for the graduate and the scholarly community since research results are unlikely to be recognised in scientific publications or comprised in comprehensive literature evaluations (Smaldone et al., 2019). It is claimed that publishing and sharing research findings are crucial for building a solid research career (Leland, 2023). As the authors' collaboration created the current book, the synergy and cooperation on the topics have developed new venues for understanding phenomena of social complexities and micro-society; the results can now be capitalised with publications to set the route to new ideas and policies in interprofessional practice (see Lehna et al. 2016). To diffuse the findings of the current book, we aim to proceed in three steps. The first step was completing the present text and proposing it to a scientific publisher. The aim was to diffuse the book's contents and use accessible language for all healthcare professionals and the general public. As discussed in the book, the keywords 'interprofessional' and 'handover' target all public and private healthcare settings. A quick guide to the topic will help them achieve teamwork, patient welfare, and value of care policies. With a book as a lever, we plan to disseminate a press release with a press agency. It will be vital to inform international interprofessional organisations by sending them a copy of the book to be advertised on their organisational web page.

Values framework

Our systemic perspective is also a different ethical standpoint for systematic research, where the researchers' and subjects' physical separation is often required for objectivist research. Instead, as practitioner-researchers, we developed insiders' knowledge of our global systems by identifying and exploring realities from this standpoint to create an 'ethics of care' (Costley and Gibbs, 2006). Nonetheless, from an ethical point of view, where needed, the public works/publications had ethics approval, except when they were theoretical studies or literature reviews. Ethics also affected the diffusion of outcomes and guided any subsequent concepts and theories from our analysis. The ethics of self-reflective practice demands that the researcher be mindful and protective of the subjects studied by defending their dignity and integrity while recognising their vulnerability (Gibbs et al., 2007). Too sectorial or biased generalisations about interprofessional team performances might hurt research organisations (Gibbs et al., 2007), which might find that the research outcomes could somehow discredit or jeopardise some organisational policies.

For instance, on one side, our research has found that there are hubs of professionals who never share information with their teams. Conversely, we know this condition might not fulfil the local and organisational requirements for clinical communication and patient safety. Shall we then disclose these findings for the sake of knowledge? How would that impact that organisation's reputation and us as researchers? Another instance is generalising results that find threats to the quality of care from specific interprofessional networks; publishing these findings can harm those teams and organisations that instead performed well but were not included in the studies or that did not reflect all the social networks emerging from our research.

The challenges we faced while drawing the conclusions from our research and suggesting MRTs were like opening Pandora's box: we were faced with the possibility that we might unlock universal meanings and find universal applicability for our findings; that we might, in other words, move from practical, middle-range ideas to grand theories. It is up to other researchers and policymakers in healthcare organisations to examine if our views of findings have hit the 'truth' or if we have entirely missed it instead.

WBL undertakings use the workplace as the setting for conducting studies, where knowledge appreciation, generation and application are vital to investigating and developing the project's methodology (Costley and Armsby, 2007b). Work on a project includes methods that enhance the practitioner's capacity to manage and generate initiatives with potential influence on their company and professional field (Costley and Armsby, 2007b). Viewed through such a perspective, our publications were similar to WBL projects.

In the current book, we explored whether the observed social networks were unique to specific situations, events and individuals or whether they could accurately reflect comparable conditions, events and people. Researchers of organisational learning might wonder, as posed by Argyris and Schön (1996), if the patterns of limited understanding they find are laws that are in some way ingrained in the structure of organisational life or if they are, in a sense, personal interpretations peculiar to the practitioners conducting the observations.

Work-based learning values and a theory of change as a middle-range theory

The following are our conclusive MRTs. The management of any healthcare organisation does not always accommodate rapid innovation and new management styles. At the same time, no identifiable person is in command of the different sub-sections where change is desired (Basole, Bodner and Rouse, 2012). Instead, as indirectly emerging from our research, various organisational value systems influence teamwork from within or outside the team. Each level is a bearer of specific and concentric values and etiquettes, such as individual, group, organisational, environmental, societal and an overarching value of WBL, which encompasses all of them (Figure 8.7.).

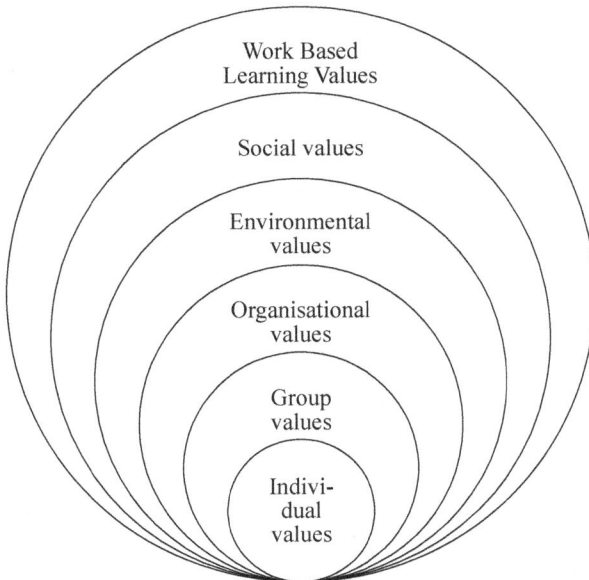

Figure 8.7. – Concentric values in WBL and interprofessional practice and change.

WBL and its value system will affect the cascade of change policies and the stakeholders' expectations.

An individual value system and change

This value level is about learning how to modulate one's own emotions, beliefs and behaviours in interprofessional teams. Though training offers workers the skills and information needed to conduct their jobs and activities effectively, it does not help create value for them (Nikolou-Walker and Meaklim, 2010). More inclusive value learning is, therefore, needed. As reported in our book chapter, *Theoretical Models of Social Mind and Social Thinking in Interprofessional Education* (Lazzari, Masiello and Shoka, 2017), emotional benefits are obtained from working collaboratively, as solo workers feel anxious about having no backup in their clinical decisions. In addition, in a cooperative interprofessional team, each professional feels empowered and encouraged to make decisions and thinks that a team provides excellent support for sharing one's findings and responsibilities and achieving common goals and values (Lazzari, Masiello and Shoka, 2017). Our future research in this direction is to understand how to implement the individual skills of building reciprocal trust and mutual understanding in addition to clinical objectives as a pathway to learning collaborative practice.

The group value system and change

This value level is about learning how to modulate collective behaviours when interprofessional practice occurs as integrated care. WBL is generally incidental and not acknowledged as a distinct learning practice; most individuals are unaware that they are acquiring new skills as part of their regular jobs (Nikolou-Walker and Lavery, 2009). Instead, knowing the direction of incidental group learning is paramount for extracting the social meaning system that shapes interprofessional values. SNA can help pull the network configuration of task distribution in healthcare settings, capture labour distribution and interprofessional standards, and detect bottlenecks in information sharing while illustrating the reinforcement points in knowledge management for better patient care (Lazzari, 2018). How interprofessional teams perform thus can be explored by ethnographically observing their behaviours and the results of their actions, extracting pervasive group values and areas of reinforcement (Lazzari, 2018). As seen, policies for healthcare settings advocate a core set of desired behaviours in multidisciplinary teams (Lazzari, 2018). Hence, the only practical method for investigating collaborative and organisational behaviours and values that healthcare administrators aim to foster in their hospitals may be an ethnographic study by participant observation (Lazzari, 2018). These 'observable behaviours' mainly occur during the teams' regular clinic practice and performances and represent the interactive goals of interprofessional practice and the shared values within groups (Lazzari, 2018).

Learning with and from others is the core skill and value in interprofessional WBL (Lazzari and Rabottini, 2021). The added values of WBL are, thus, linked to specific processes occurring in organisations, such as (1) participating in group activities, (2) collaborating with others, (3) reflecting, attending and watching others, (4) offering and accepting any feedback from teammates, and (5) shadowing and being supervised (Eraut, 2011). Improved team collaboration has a cascade effect on the quality of the service and patient satisfaction. We found how patients could recognise and appreciate when they receive integrated care from interprofessional teams (Lazzari and Masiello, 2017). Therefore, the group value system extends to incorporate, merge, safeguard and improve customers' standards of care and satisfaction as the two system values (patients' and teams') work as an integrated force (Lazzari, 2004). When interprofessional practice is successful, the customers attended to by these teams also record increased satisfaction with the care they receive (Lazzari and Masiello, 2017); they can distinguish when an interprofessional team is operating and when it is not (Lazzari, McAleer and Rabottini, 2022). An improved collaborative approach can thus reduce complaints from patients and their families, who frequently report to the hospital managers that their allocated care teams provide fragmentary care (Lazzari and Masino, 2015). In such cases, no harmonisation exists between primary and secondary care and HCPs about the agreed-upon plans for a specific patient (Lazzari and Masiello, 2017). Our future research in this direction will measure the degree of co-variation between patients' satisfaction and interprofessional team collaboration.

The organisational value system and change

This value system occurs when healthcare organisations learn how to promote inclusion and non-discrimination policies in teamwork and buffer inequalities and group conflicts or disparities. A health organisation is a higher-order system that affects lower-order systems and interprofessional dynamics—directly inside the hospitals and wards. Linking educational talents with actual circumstances takes hypotheses and conjectures out of the classroom into an organisation, store, or wherever people *develop and apply knowledge* (Nikolou-Walker, 2007). This process of WBL applied to interprofessional teams sees each team member exchanging information and feedback about patients among the team; interprofessional social systems can accomplish their organisational goals, adhere to clinical governance and remain operative as a living and value-based social system by learning from successes or failures (Lazzari, 2004). As highlighted in our book *The Assessment of Interprofessional Learning and Practice in Psychiatry* (Lazzari and Rabottini, 2021), team building, collaborative care, WBL and interprofessional communication can occur when health carers as learners are provided with feedback about the outcomes of their interprofessional practice. This feedback derives from colleagues, the organisation, families, or accessing targeted teaching or real-time feedback (Lazzari and Rabottini, 2021). With the support of ad-hoc CPD courses and clear organisational policies, this process of cogwheel-integrated social systems can increase professionals' mindfulness (Lazzari and Rabottini, 2021). The benefit is that HCPs become aware of the risk of creating hubs or sub-teams of co-workers from the same professional background while excluding equally important 'ancillary' professionals during patient handover and care (Lazzari and Rabottini, 2021). We have shown that a supportive healthcare organisation can address the risk of less-than-optimal interprofessional practice. Moreover, successful teamwork can mend communication flow and professional malpractice blockages. Our future research in this direction will use SNA to capture how interprofessional communication during handover impacts on treatment value and patient wellbeing.

The environmental value system and changes

This value level is about empowering the ancillary departments of healthcare that support better work organisations and teamwork by involving outsourcing training and regulatory bodies external to the wards or hospitals. Regional policies and national regulations should reinforce the human resources department to advocate for reasonable shifts, effective office setups and functioning technology. Policies are also vital to regulate work well-being and stress reduction. Attention should also be provided to interpersonal proxemics, considering how overcrowded and unhealthy offices affect team dynamics. At other times, line managers need to redesign their teams and make efforts to select people who will naturally collaborate—knowing that people who have a propensity to conflict with teammates might destabilise the whole organisation. According to a constructivist approach, this (tacit) knowledge (and wisdom) can be actively constructed through learning (Nikolou-Walker and Curley, 2011).

The environmental change also includes regional, national or international task forces to promote interprofessional practice and make it an inspiration for healthcare systems in different countries. As reported in one of our earliest books on work ethics, *Psychology and Ethics of Works and Organisations*, the motivation to improve by emulating what 'more successful teams do' is always strong in healthcare settings (Lazzari, 2004). Being open to environmental values is about breaking the boundaries of regional or local ways of doing things. When seen under a systemic lens, organisations might naturally become impenetrable by environmental/external values and influences (by increasing their entropy) (Lazzari and Rabottini, 2021). Some teams or hospitals might be unaware of regional and international regulatory bodies that have set general principles of interprofessional practice.

On the contrary, being open to external scrutiny and assessment is necessary for quality certification in the UK (see CQC, 2022). Another book, *The Psychology and Ethics of Companies and Corporate Relations*, highlights the risk of locked social systems in the organisation when they do not interact collaboratively with their environment (Lazzari, 2006). As we mentioned earlier in the systemic theory, the risk of prejudiced organisations is to become self-referenced in their value system (Lazzari, 2006). These protected organisations might allegedly progress adrift, adopting exclusive corporate identities and work ethics (Lazzari, 2006). Self-referencing organisations and corporations that do not adapt to collaborative values often can conflict with what is recommended by the professional bodies' policies—for example, the Royal College of Nursing, the Committee for Quality and Care (CQC), the General Medical Council, the Nurse and Midwifery Council and the British Psychological Society (Lazzari, 2006). In these conditions, change becomes challenging. Our future research in this direction is to extract a dataset of several healthcare organisations investigated for incidents in interprofessional practice.

The societal value system and change
This value system empowers and protects healthcare organisations and interprofessional teams to deal with complex cases or patients. Sometimes, teams receive complaints from 'service users, their families or colleagues' regarding the service and care provided. When a complaint is made, the team can feel threatened in its harmony. Right or wrong, team members under the pressure of external investigations for allegedly professional negligence or patients' complaints might start to split and diverge in their priorities or opinions. Professionally, these moments should generate self-reflective practice and learning from errors. WBL and reflective practice should be closely related and complementary, changing how workplace and work experience are perceived and regulated (Nikolou-Walker and Garnett, 2004). Redesigning social networks in healthcare organisations should use information flow and knowledge management as a dynamic and constant lever for exchanging information from the central hubs of practitioners to the peripheral ones in patient care and community teams (Lazzari, 2018).

Such a redesign will reinforce interprofessional bonds to the advantage of the treatment values and patient well-being. The society, identifiable by organisational or internal clients (health carers and healthcare organisations) and societal or external clients (patients, service users and their families, community healthcare teams), is a complex network of mingled and interacting individuals who constantly dialogue by sharing information, plans, resources and expectations (Lazzari and Masiello, 2016). In our book, *Communication Neurosciences for Interprofessional Teams in Health Care* (Lazzari and Masiello, 2016), we suggest that social interactions among interprofessional team members and between them and their service users/patients are regulated by our social brain. In other words, interpersonal behaviours are normalised by our mind, which has specific skills that help us interact with other humans, interpret social cues, act as prosocial individuals, predict our and others' behaviours, and use empathy to unite with others (Lazzari and Masiello, 2016).

For example, older adults who live socially isolated because of the COVID-19 pandemic are more at risk of dementia due to a lack of opportunities for social interactions (Lazzari and Rabottini, 2022). Therefore, complex brain mechanisms help humans integrate their emotions, behaviours, actions and communication; our brains, it is believed, are built in such a way as to allow our social interactions, and we act socially and interprofessionaly also because our brains have had an evolutionary development to help us live and thrive within the social systems where we are located (Lazzari, 2007; Lazzari and Masiello, 2016). Our future research in this direction is to use neurophysiological parameters (e.g., consensual/group EEG, ECG, blood pressure) to capture interprofessional interactions and confirm the experimental hypothesis that interprofessional practice is 'also' supported by complex neurophysiological networks in our (social) brain (Lazzari and Masiello, 2016).

The education of WBL values and changes
This value level is about improving the flow of learning in teams; it allows moments of promoting and sharing the humanistic meanings of participatory care at reflective meetings, where team members can explore the unspoken and unseen aspects of their work in the team (Costley, Nottingham and Nikolou-Walker, 2021). However, there is a need to provide more room in WBL for tacit, unforeseen learning and to include more humanistic elements of knowledge that contribute to effective business practices (Costley, Nottingham and Nikolou-Walker, 2021). Consequently, corporate goals might also be attained by educating healthcare professionals to understand and reinforce their ethical bonds

and strengthening their competencies for mutual understanding and support (Lazzari, 2004). Reflective practice is one of the instruments of investigation used in WBL and work-based research (Siebert and Costley, 2013). Reflection as a learning method allows practitioners to contest presumptions about their jobs, which incites employees to query the values that guide their work (Siebert and Costley, 2013). However, the value of advanced WBL to businesses seems to depend on how well the workplace can accommodate workers experiencing fast personal and professional growth (Lester and Costley, 2010).

In our research on organisations and interprofessional practice, sometimes, we have found gaps in interpersonal value systems and missing educational moments to learn cooperatively. Some teams integrated well and applied the required skills to communicate with their team members and patients, with a reciprocal effect between the two and using interpersonal skills correctly (Lazzari, Gandolfi-Colleoni and Trallo, 1996). On the other hand, other settings appeared less focused on cooperative participation and care as they had different goals that did not require shared objectives (Lazzari, 1997). Where, then, to learn interprofessional skills and modus operandi? Universities remain the leading organisation for certifying, approving and investigating any aspect of interprofessional practice, especially if courses are linked to clinical departments. However, it is possible to make the case that despite these parameters, the university's role as the accrediting agency still makes it the investing and controlling organisation; as a result, the most prominent value schemes are those incorporated in the school's conceptual structures and apparatus (Armsby, Costley and Jonathan, 2006). Yet, a collaboration between healthcare organisations and the academy is the ideal.

Our early ideas about promoting interprofessional practice and ethics in organisational relations and healthcare learners were derived from unobtrusive and ethnographic observations of team challenges in public hospitals (Lazzari, 2014). The study showed that interprofessional value conflicts could eventually influence agreed-upon targets and have a cascading and unpredictable impact on patient care (Lazzari, 2004). In contrast, we observed that undergraduate interprofessional students show increased satisfaction with learning interprofessional skills and the strategies of mutual support; they feel that they can apply collaborative skills in their routine clinical practice by utilising interpersonal kindness, empathy and active listening (Lazzari and Masiello, 2017b). Their interprofessional education made them more aware of the value of and potential support from the other HCPs in their teams with different areas of expertise (Lazzari and Masiello, 2017b). A significant lever for change is the personal feeling of agency and empowerment, believing that change in work ethics is possible and achievable by small but significant steps.

Our future research in this direction will use education to promote WBL values and interprofessional practice by creating a hybrid combination of approved university courses in interprofessional training and continuing professional development (CPD) modules. A short online module on basic interprofessional concepts to communicate with many busy healthcare professionals and collect some information about their practice is also predicted.

Towards a plan of implementation

The current book has adhered to the present trends in EBP. More medically oriented policymakers pursue a quality and safety improvement route in which care systems are thoroughly assessed for error and failure and then corrected by workplace-based, multi-professional groups (Zwarenstein and Reeves, 2006). Implementing our observations is a required step to disseminate our MRTs. The term 'implement' originates from the Latin *implere*, which means to achieve or apply; as a result, research focusing on the application is a scientific enquiry about achievements (Rhydderch, 2004; Peters et al., 2019). The implementation aims to transform an intention into accomplishment, which in health research can be guidelines, plans or distinct performances (jointly called policies) with observable modifications—applications and healthcare plans make visible and practical modifications of the current (interprofessional) practice and procedures (Rhydderch, 2004; Peters et al., 2019). Our healthcare research goal was to answer questions and solve problems (Polit and Beck, 2022) about current and applicative stages of interprofessional practice.

A significant area of medical management aims to generate directives and stability (Swanwick and McKimm, 2010) in health organisations by disentangling organisational obstacles and directing people (Covey et al., 1994). The management areas where health organisations require great attention and where we will focus our future research efforts are as follows: (1) organisational design and the provision of technical and human supplies, (2) management that specifies corporate configuration and creates institutional guidelines, and (3) the supervision and solving of challenges, such as producing original solutions (Northouse, 2004). Hays (2012) states that leadership comprises three roles: governance, management and training. One of the difficulties with work-based initiatives for academic objectives is that they might develop into academic constructs that are not always well-integrated into working practices (Costley and Abukari, 2015). Even when used widely, projects could be merely one of the activities employees participate in (Costley and Abukari, 2015). Instead, work-based developments might provide a 'snapshot' of a person's or a group of people's capacities to innovate, transform or enhance a working environment (Costley and Abukari, 2015). Work-based projects provide the chance to (1) dig into a hypothetical and speculative realm, (2) conduct a study and development utilising a thorough and methodical methodology, and (3) realise a variety of potential routes and working practice options (Costley and Abukari, 2015).

Our next steps in this area will be to establish online courses for healthcare professionals to enhance their awareness of interprofessional communication and practice and make them mindful of the consequences of collaborative care on patient care and safety. However, as we aim to promote awareness, self-reflective practice and learning, we will strive to make these learning processes attractive and objective based on a few fundamental signposts of interprofessional care.

Limitations of the book

Though we engaged in meta-cognition or internal supervision that enabled us to be self-aware during our interaction with others, we also realised that we sometimes acknowledged some insights quickly.

There were other intuitions about a better quality of care and interprofessional practice that we did not recognise easily, deriving from the characteristics of the interactions or the typology of interpersonal and interprofessional conflicts. At times, the familiarity with a setting or team did not allow us sufficient scientific detachment to capture salient points of interprofessional teams that were not sharable among different environments.

Reaching a broader perspective on our area of interprofessional research required more control to ensure that we were not too biased by our familiarity or normalisation of the observed behaviours deriving from prolonged exposure and scientifically unsupervised studies about these social conditions (Ferguson, 2018). Furthermore, our risk of participating in interprofessional teams was that we could become defensive about gaps in our research instruments, which could decrease the impact of our self-reflective practice and distort thinking and feeling (Ferguson, 2018)—for example, struggling to find a boundary between our direct participation into interprofessional teams and having sufficient detachment to explore these settings objectively.

Additionally, failure to increase interprofessional cooperation will result from the unconsidered use of interactive technology with no approval by the team to reach an understanding of successful exchange and a shared viewpoint on cooperation (Müller et al., 2018). However, the outcomes of this book are consistent with theories of groundbreaking settings as having a visibly stated idea, a safe atmosphere for qualified growth and scholarship, a collective awareness of interprofessional values and collaborative perspectives, hands-on assistance and a chance to pioneer and promote innovative practices (West and Farr, 1990) (Figure 8.8.).

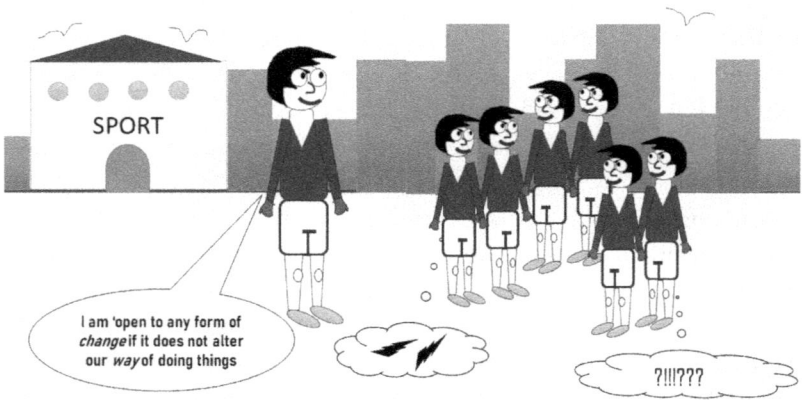

Figure 8.8. – Change plans agreed in teams need to review positions of power that can facilitate or hinder the whole process.

References

American Speech-Language-Hearing Association (2023). Evidence-Based Practice. Webpage]. Available at: https://www.asha.org/research/ (Accessed: 29 March 2023).

Anderson, C. R. and McLachlan, S. (2015) 'Transformative research as knowledge mobilization: Transmedia, bridges, and layers', *Action Research*, 14(3), pp. 295–317. Available at: https://doi.org/10.1177/1476750315616684 (Accessed: 20 February 2022).

Andrade, H. and Valtcheva, A. (2009) 'Promoting learning and achievement through self-assessment', *Theory Into Practice*, 48(1), pp. 12–19. Available at: https://doi.org/10.1080/00405840802577544 (Accessed: 20 February 2022).

Anonymous (2008). *Higher education governance in Europe*. Brussels: Eurydice European Unit. Available at: www.eurydice.org.

Anonymous. Quote by Albert Einstein: 'Not everything that can be counted counts and n...' (goodreads.com)

APA Dictionary Online (2023). Ecological validity. [Online]. Available at: https://dictionary.apa.org/ecological-validity (Accessed: 7 April 2023).

APA, American Psychological Association (2013). Definition of evidence-based practice. [Online]. Available at: https://dictionary.apa.org/evidence-based-practice

APA, American Psychological Association (no date) *Apa Dictionary of Psychology, American Psychological Association*. American Psychological Association. Available at: https://dictionary.apa.org/thick-description (Accessed: March 26, 2023).

Argyris, C. and Schön, D. A. (1974) *Theory in practice: Increasing professional effectiveness*. San Francisco, CA: Jossy-Bass Publishers.

Argyris, C. and Schön, D. A. (1996) *Organizational learning II: Theory, method, and practice.* Wokingham, England: Addison-Wesley.

Armsby, P. Costley, C. and Garnett, J. (2006) 'The legitimisation of knowledge: A work-based learning perspective of APEL', *International Journal of Lifelong Education*, 25(4), pp. 369–383. Available at: https://doi.org/10.1080/02601370600772368 (Accessed: 7 April 2023).

Australian Medical Association. (2007). *Guidance on clinical handover.* [online] Available at: https://www.ama.com.au/article/guidance-clinical-handover.

Bandura, A. (1971) *Social learning theory.* New York: General Learning Press.

Barr, H. et al. (2015) *Effective interprofessional education.* Oxford: Blackwell Publishing.

Barr, H. et al. (2016) 'Steering the development of interprofessional education', *Journal of Interprofessional Care*, 30(5), pp. 549–552. Available at: https://doi.org/10.1080/13561820.2016.1217686 (Accessed: 7 June 2021).

Bartgis, J., and Bigfoot, D. (2010). Healthy Indian Country Initiative Promising Prevention Practices Resource Guide. National Indian Health Board Edition, Healthy Indian Country Initiative Promising Prevention Practices Resource Guide. (Online) Available at: https://www.nihb.org/docs/04072010/2398_NIHB%20HICI%20Book_web.pdf

Basole, R. C., Bodner, D. A. and Rouse, W. B. (2012) 'Healthcare management through organisational simulation', *Decision Support Systems*, 55(2), pp. 552–563. Available at: https://doi.org/10.1016/j.dss.2012.10.012 (Accessed: 5 May 2022).

Bassot, B. (2016) *The reflective practice guide.* London: Routledge.

Bazaluk, O. (2017) 'Plato's and Isocrates' traditions in the development of educational theories in the history of culture', *Annals of the University of Craiova–Philosophy Series*, 40(2), pp. 5–18. Available at: ResearchGate (Accessed: 5 May 2022).

Beard, K. S. (2015) 'Theoretically speaking: An interview with Mihaly Csikszentmihalyi on flow theory development and its usefulness in addressing contemporary challenges in education', *Educational Psychological Review*, 27, pp. 353–364. Available at: https://doi.org/10.1007/s10648-014-9291-1 (Accessed: 5 May 2022).

Belbase, S., Luitel, B. and Taylor, P. (2013) 'Autoethnography: A method of research and teaching for transformative education', *Journal of Education and Research*, 1(1), pp. 86–95. Available at: https://www.learntechlib.org/p/208799/ (Accessed: 20 April 2022).

Black P. and William D. (2008) 'Assessment and classroom learning', *Assessment in Education*, 5(1), pp. 7–74. Available at: http://dx.doi.org/10.1080/0969595980050102 (Accessed: 20 April 2022).

Bleakley, A. (1999) 'From reflective practice to holistic reflexivity', *Studies in Higher Education*, 24(3), pp. 315–330. Available at: http://doi.org/10.1080/03075079912331379925 (Accessed: 10 February 2022).

Bonell, C., Oakley, A., Hargreaves, J., Strange, V. and Rees, R. (2006) 'Assessment of generalisability in trials of health interventions: suggested framework and systematic review', *BMJ*, 333(7563), pp. 346–349. Available at: https://doi.org/10.1136/bmj.333.7563.346 (Accessed: 7 April 2023).

Breen, D., O'Brien, S., McCarthy, N., Gallagher, A. and Walshe, N. (2019) 'Effect of a proficiency-based progression simulation programme on clinical communication for the deteriorating patient: a randomised controlled trial', *BMJ Open*, 9(7), p.e025992. Available at: https://doi.org/10.1136/bmjopen-2018-025992 (Accessed: 7 April 2023).

Bridges, D. R. et al. (2011) 'Interprofessional collaboration: Three best practice models of interprofessional education', *Medical Education Online*, 16, pp. 1–10. Available at: https://doi.org/10.3402/meo.v16io.6035 (Accessed: 3 April 2022).

British Psychological Society [BPS] (2017). *Practice Guideline,* 3rd Ed. London: British Psychological Society. Available at: https://www.bps.org.uk/guideline/bps-practice-guidelines-2017-0 (Accessed: 15 June 2022).

Budworth, T., Al Hashemi, S. G. and Waddah, S. G. (2015) *Reflective learning.* London: Routledge-CRC Press. Kindle Edition.

Burchett, H., Umoquit, M. and Dobrow, M. (2011) 'How do we know when research from one setting can be useful in another? A review of external validity, applicability and transferability frameworks', *Journal of Health Services Research Policy*,16(4): pp. 238–44. Available at: https://doi.org/10.1258/jhsrp.2011.010124 (Accessed: 15 June 2022).

Burgess, A., van Diggele, C., Roberts, C. and Mellis, C. (2020) 'Teaching Clinical Handover With ISBAR', *BMC Medical Education*, [online] 20(2), pp.1–8. Available at: https://doi.org/10.1186/s12909-020-02285-0 (Accessed: 15 June 2022).

Buron, B. (2008) 'Levels of personhood: A model for dementia care', *Geriatric Nursing*, 29(5), pp. 324–332. Available at: https://doi. org/10.1016/j.gerinurse.2007.11.001 (Accessed: 1 April 2022).

Cambridge Dictionary Online (2022) *System*. Available at: https:// dictionary.cambridge.org/dictionary/english/system (Accessed: 20 April 2022)

Campbell, H., Hotchkiss, R., Bradshaw, N. and Porteous, M. (1998) 'Integrated care pathways', *BMJ*, 316(133). Available at: https://doi. org/10.1136/bmj.316.7125.133 (Accessed: 20 May 2022).

Care Quality Commission (CQC) (2022) *Our purpose and role*. Available at: https://www.cqc.org.uk/about-us/our-purpose-role/who-we-are (Accessed: 20 May 2022).

Care Quality Commission (CQC) (2022). *Golden standards*. [Website]. Available at: https://www.cqc.org.uk/guidance-providers/healthcare/ management-information-good (Accessed: 20 May 2022).

Carminati, L. (2018) 'Generalizability in Qualitative Research: A Tale of Two Traditions', *Qualitative Health Research*; 28(13): pp. 2094–2101. Available at: https://doi.org/10.1177/1049732318788379 (Accessed: 8 April 2022).

Carona, C., Handford, C. and Fonseca, A. (2021) 'Socratic questioning put into clinical practice', *British Journal of Psychiatry Advances*, 27(6), pp. 424–426. Available at: https://doi.org/10.1192/bja.2020.77 (Accessed: 8 April 2022).

Chang, H., (2013) 'Individual and collaborative autoethnography as method', in Jones, S. H., Adams, T. A. and Ellis, C. (eds.) *Handbook of autoethnography*. London: Routledge, pp.107–122.

Clark, T., Foster, L., Sloan, L. and Bryman, A. (2021) *Bryman's social research methods*. Oxford: Oxford University Press.

Collis, J. and Hussey, R. (2017) *Business research* (p. 46). City: Macmillan Education UK.

Conn, L.G., Lingard, L., Reeves, S., Miller, K.-L., Russell, A. and Zwarenstein, M. (2009) 'Communication Channels in General Internal Medicine: A Description of Baseline Patterns for Improved Interprofessional Collaboration', *Qualitative Health Research*, 19(7), pp. 943–953. Available at: https://doi.org/10.1177/1049732309338282 (Accessed: 23 September 2022).

Costley, C. and Abukari, A. (2015) 'The impact of work-based research projects at postgraduate level', *Journal of Work-Applied Management*, 7(1), pp. 3–14. Available at: www.emeraldinsight.com/2205-2062.htm (Accessed: 23 September 2022).

Costley, C. and Armsby, P. (2007a) 'Research influences on a professional doctorate', *Research in Post-Compulsory Education*, 12(3), pp. 343–355. Available at: https://doi.org/10.1080/13596740701559803 (Accessed: 13 April 2022).

Costley, C. and Armsby, P. (2007b) 'Work-based learning assessed as a field or a mode of study', *Assessment and Evaluation in Higher Education*, 32(1), pp. 21–33. Available at: https://doi.org/10.1080/02602930600848267 (Accessed: 13 April 2022).

Costley, C. and Dikerdem, M.A., (2011) *Work based learning pedagogies and academic development*. Project Report. Middlesex University, London, UK. [Monograph]

Costley, C. and Fulton, J. (eds.) (2018) *Methodologies for practice research: Approaches for professional doctorates*. London: Sage.

Costley, C. and Gibbs, G. (2006) 'Researching others: Care as an ethic for practitioner researchers', *Studies in Higher Education*, 31(1), pp. 89–98, Available at: https://doi.org/10.1080/03075070500392375 (Accessed: 13 June 2022).

Costley, C., Elliott, G. C. and Gibbs, P. (2010) *Doing work-based research: Approaches to enquiry for insider-researchers*. London: SAGE.

Costley, C., Nottingham, P. and Nikolou-Walker, E. (2021) 'Equality, diversity and inclusion for work and learning in higher education', *Work Based Learning e-Journal*, 10(2), pp. 42–52. Available at: https://wblearning-ejournal.com/uploads/text_with_images/3.1wledicolloquiumbriefingpaper1639773424.pdf (Accessed: 13 April 2022).

Crossley, N. (2008) 'Social networks and student activism: On the politicising effect of campus connections', *The Sociological Review*, 56(1), pp. 18–38. Available at: https://doi.org/10.1111%2Fj.1467-954X.2008.00775.x (Accessed: 13 April 2022).

Crossley, N., Bellotti, E., Edwards, G., Everett, M. G., Koskinen, J. and Tranmer, M. (2015) *Social network analysis for ego-nets*. Los Angeles, CA: SAGE.

Csikszentmihalyi, M. (1990) *Flow: The psychology of optimal experience*. New York: Harper and Row.

Csikszentmihalyi, M. (1997) 'Assessing aesthetic education: Measuring the ability to "ward off chaos"', *Arts Education Policy Review*, 99(1), pp. 33–38. Available at: https://doi.org/10.1080/10632919709600763 (Accessed: 10 February 2022).

Cunningham, F. C. et al. (2012) 'Health professional networks as a vector for improving healthcare quality and safety: A systematic review', *BMJ Quality and Safety* 21(3), pp. 239–249. Available at: https://doi.org/10.1136/bmjqs-2011-000187 (Accessed: 10 February 2022).

Curran, V. et al. (2012) 'An approach to integrating interprofessional education in collaborative mental health care', *Academic Psychiatry*, 36(2), pp. 91–95. Available at: https://doi.org/10.1176/appi.ap.10030045 (Accessed: 10 March 2022).

Custer, D. (2014) 'Autoethnography as a transformative research method', *The Qualitative Report*, 19(37), pp. 1–13. Available at: http://citeseerx.ist.psu.edu/viewdoc/download?doi=10.1.1.852.573andrep=rep1andtype=pdf (Accessed: 10 March 2022).

Dawes, M., Summerskill, W., Glasziou, P. *et al.* (2005) 'Sicily statement on evidence-based practice', *BMC Medical Education*, 5, 1. Available at: https://doi.org/10.1186/1472-6920-5-1 (Accessed: 10 March 2022).

de Gans, S., Penturij-Kloks, M., Scheele, F., van de Pol, M., van der Zwaard. B. and Keijsers, C. (2022) 'Combined *inter*professional and *intra*professional clinical collaboration reduces length of stay and consultations: a retrospective cohort study on an intensive collaboration ward (ICW)', *Journal of Interprofessional Care*, 1(9). doi: 10.1080/13561820.2022.2137117. (Accessed: 10 March 2022).

Decety, J. and Steinbeis, N. (2020) 'Multiple mechanisms of prosocial development,' in Decety, J. (ed.), *The social brain: A developmental perspective*. London: The MIT Press.

Delle Fave, A. and Massimi, F. (2005) 'The relevance of subjective well-being to social policies: Optimal experience and tailored intervention', in Huppert F., Keverne B. and Baylis N. (eds), *The science of well-being*. Oxford: Oxford University Press.

Delle Fave, A., Massimi, F. and Bassi, M. (2011) *Psychological selection and optimal experience across cultures*. Dordrecht, Heidelberg, London, New York: Springer.

Dingley, C. et al. (2008) 'Improving patient safety through provider communication strategy enhancements', in Henriksen K. et al. (eds.) *Advances in patient safety: New directions and alternative approaches (Vol. 3: Performance and tools)*. Rockville (MD): Agency for Healthcare Research and Quality (US). Available at: https://www.ncbi.nlm.nih.gov/books/NBK43671/?report=reader

Eggins, S. and Slade, D. (2015) 'Communication in clinical handover: Improving the safety and quality of the patient experience', *Journal of Public Health Research*, 4(3). Available at: https://doi.org/10.4081/jphr.2015.666 (Accessed: 1 May 2022).

Ellaway, R. and Masters, K. (2008) 'AMEE guide 32: e-Learning in medical education Part 1: Learning, teaching and assessment', *Medical Teacher*, 30(5): pp. 455–473. Available at: https://doi.org/10.1080/01421590802108331 (Accessed: 1 May 2021).

Ellis, C., Adams, T. E. and Bochner, A. P. (2011) 'Autoethnography: An overview', *Historical Social Research / Historische Sozialforschung*, 36(4 (138)), pp. 273–290. Available at: http://www.jstor.org/stable/23032294 (Accessed: 10 February 2022).

Encyclopaedia Britannica (2022) *Epistemology*. Available at: https://www.britannica.com/topic/epistemology (Accessed: 8 April 2022).

Encyclopaedia Britannica (2022) *Ethnography*. Available at: https://www.britannica.com/science/ethnography (Accessed: 8 April 2022).

Eraut, M. (2011) 'Informal learning in the workplace: Evidence on the real value of work-based learning (WBL).' *Development and Learning in Organizations: An International Journal*, 25(5), pp. 8–12. Available at: https://doi.org/10.1108/14777281111159375 (Accessed: 1 October 2022).

Fazio, S., Pace, D., Flinner, J. and Kallourer, B. (2018) 'The fundamentals of person-centered care for individuals with dementia', *The Gerontologist*, 58(1), pp. S10–S19. Available at: https://doi.org/10.1093/geront/gnx122 (Accessed: 5 April 2022).

Ferenczi, S. (1994) *Final contributions to the problems and methods of psycho-analysis*. London: Karnac Books.

Ferguson, H. (2018) 'How social workers reflect in action and when and why they don't: The possibilities and limits to reflective practice in social work', *Social Work Education*, 37(4), pp. 415–427. Available at: https://doi.org/10.1080/02615479.2017.1413083 (Accessed: 5 April 2022).

Ferguson, L. (2004) 'External validity, generalizability, and knowledge utilization', *Journal of Nursing Scholarship*, 36(1), pp. 16–22. Available at: https://doi.org/10.1111/j.1547-5069.2004.04006.x (Accessed: 4 May 2022)

Finch, J. (2000) 'Interprofessional education and teamworking: A view from the education providers', *BMJ*, 321(7269), pp. 1138–1140. Available at: https://doi.org/10.1136/bmj.321.7269.1138 (Accessed: 8 April 2022).

Fiorella, L. and Mayer, R. (2013) 'The relative benefits of learning by teaching and teaching expectancy', *Contemporary Educational Psychology*, 28, pp. 281–288. Available at: https://dx.doi.org/10.1016/j.cedpsych.2013.06.001 (Accessed: 1 June 2022).

Fook, J. (2018) 'Reflective models and frameworks in practice', in Costley, C. and Fulton, J. (eds.) *Methodologies for practice research: Approaches for professional doctorates*. London: Sage.

Foronda, C., MacWilliams, B. and McArthur, E. (2016) 'Interprofessional communication in healthcare: An integrative review', *Nurse Education in Practice*, 19, pp. 36–40. Available at: https://doi.org/10.1016/j.nepr.2016.04.005 (Accessed: 5 July 2022).

Fraser, S. A. and Greenhalgh, T. (2001) 'Coping with complexity', *BMJ*, 323(7316), pp. 799–803. Available at: https://doi.org/10.1136/bmj.323.7316.799 (Accessed: 21 April 2022).

Frenk, J. et al. (2010) 'Health professionals for a new century: Transforming education to strengthen health systems in an interdependent world', *The Lancet*, 376(9756), pp. 1923–1958. Available at: https://doi.org/10.1016/s0140-6736(10)61854-5 (Accessed: 3 April 2022).

Fuhse, J. A. (2015) 'Theorizing social networks: The relational sociology of and around Harrison White', *International Review of Sociology*, 25(1), pp. 15–44. Available at: https://doi.org/10.1080/03906701.2014.997968 (Accessed: 28 May 2022).

Fulton, J., Kuit, J., Sanders, G. and Smith, P. (2019) *The professional doctorate*, London: McMillan International and Red Globe Press.

Gabbay, J. and Le May, A., (2010) *Practice-based evidence for healthcare: clinical mindlines*. London: Routledge.

General Medical Council (GMC) (2017) *An inter-professional learning scheme for medical students.* Available at: Achieving good medical practice: guidance for medical students – GMC (gmc-uk.org) (Accessed: 05 June 2022).

General Medical Council (GMC) (2018) *Communication complaint types and contributory factors report.* London: General Medical Council. Available at: communication-complaint-types-and-contributory-factors-report_pdf-80571206.pdf (gmc-uk.org) (Accessed: 24 April 2022).

General Medical Council (GMC) (2021) *Good Medical Practice.* London: General Medical Council, Available at: https://www.gmc-uk.org/ethical-guidance/ethical-guidance-for-doctors/good-medical-practice (Accessed: 15 December 2022).

General Medical Council (GMC) (2022a) *Working with colleagues.* Available at: https://www.gmc-uk.org/ethical-guidance/ethical-guidance-for-doctors/leadership-and-management-for-all-doctors/working-with-colleagues theory (Accessed: 24 April 2022).

General Medical Council (GMC) (2022b) *Domain 3: Communication partnership and teamwork.* Available at: https://www.gmc-uk.org/ethical-guidance/ethical-guidance-for-doctors/good-medical-practice/domain-3---communication-partnership-and-teamwork (Accessed: 05 June 2022).

Germain, C.P. (2001) 'Ethnography: The method', in Munhall, P. L. (ed.), *Nursing research: A qualitative perspective* (3rd ed.). National League for Nursing. Boston: Jones and Bartlett.

Gibbons, M., Limoges, C., Nowortny, H., Schwartzman, S., Scott, P. and Trow, M. (1994) *The new production of knowledge,* London, Sage.

Gibbs, P., Costley, C., Armsby, P. and Trakakis, A. (2007) 'Developing the ethics of worker-researchers through phronesis', *Teaching in Higher Education,* 12(3), pp. 365–375. Available at: https://doi.org/10.1080/13562510701278716 (Accessed: 25 May 2022).

Gibson, B. (2022) 'Systems theory', *Encyclopaedia Britannica.* Available at: https://www.britannica.com/topic/systems-theory (Accessed: 24 April 2022).

Gleeson, L., O'Brien, G.L., O'Mahony, D. and Byrne, S., (2022) 'Interprofessional communication in the hospital setting: a systematic review of the qualitative literature.' *Journal of Interprofessional Care*, 37(2), pp.1–11. Available at: https://doi.org/10.1080/13561820.2022.20 28746 (Accessed: 24 April 2022).

GMC, General Medical Council (2009). *Tomorrow's Doctors*. [Online]. Available at: GMC (Accessed: 24 April 2022).

Goffman, E. (1961) *Encounters: Two studies in the sociology of interaction*. Oxford: Bobbs-Merrill.

Goffman, E. (1963a) *Behaviour in public places: Notes on the social organisation*. New York: The Free Press.

Goffman, E. (1963b) *Stigma*. London: Penguin.

Goffman, E. (1969) *Strategic Interaction*. Philadelphia: University of Pennsylvania Press.

Goodwin, M. S., Velicer, W. F. and Intille, S. S. (2008) 'Telemetric monitoring in the behaviour sciences', *Behavior Research Methods*, 40(1), pp. 328–341. Available at: https://doi.org/10.3758/brm.40.1.328 (Accessed: 4 February 2021).

Government of Western Australia Department of Health. Clinical handover [Internet]. WA Health, Government of Western Australia. [cited 2022Dec23]. Available from: https://ww2.health.wa.gov.au/Articles/A_E/Clinical-handover

Gravem, S. A. et al. (2017) 'Transformative research is not easily predicted', *Trends in Ecology & Evolution*, 32(11), pp. 825–834. Available at: https://doi.org/10.1016/j.tree.2017.08.012 (Accessed: 21 May 2022).

Green, L.W. (2008) 'Making research relevant: if it is an evidence-based practice, where's the practice-based evidence?', *Family practice*, 25(suppl_1), pp.i20–i24. Available at: https://doi.org/10.1093/fampra/cmn055 (Accessed: 25 April 2022).

Grippa, F. et al. (2018) 'Measuring information exchange and brokerage capacity of healthcare teams', *Management Decision*. 56(10), pp. 2239–2251. Available at: https://doi.org/10.1108/MD-10-2017-1001 (Accessed: 25 April 2022).

Guba E. and Lincoln Y. (1989) *Fourth generation evaluation*. Newbury Park, CA: Sage.

Hayes, C. and Fulton, J. (2015) 'Autoethnography as a method of facili- tating critical reflexivity for professional doctorate students,' *Journal of Learning Development in Higher Education*, 8 (3), pp. 1-15. ISSN 1759-667X

Hays, J. M. and Kim, C. C. (2012) *Transforming leadership for the 21st century*. Xlibris.

Hébert, C. (2015) 'Knowing and/or experiencing: 'A critical examination of the reflective models of John Dewey and Donald Schön', *Reflective Practice*, 16(3), pp. 361–371. Available at: https://doi.org/10.1080/146239 43.2015.1023281 (Accessed: 15 February 2022).

Holifield, D., Chisholm, C., & Harris, M. (2008). 'Continuous profes- sional development by work based learning for engineers: Utilising the integration of tacit and explicit knowledge', *International Journal of Technology and Engineering Education*, 5(2), 23–30.

Holifield, M.D., Clarke, T. and Jones, E. (2011) 'Sustainability of knowledge within organisations', *Management of Sustainable Development*, 3(2).

Holmqvist, R., Philips, B. and Barkham, M. (2015) 'Developing practice-based evidence: Benefits, challenges, and tensions', *Psychotherapy Research*, 25(1), pp. 20–31. Available at: https://doi. org/10.1080/10503307.2013.861093 (Accessed: 15 February 2022).

Horn, S.D. and Gassaway, J. (2010) 'Practice based evidence: Incorporating clinical heterogeneity and patient-reported outcomes for comparative effectiveness research', *Medical Care*, Vol. 48, No. 6, Supplement 1: Comparative Effectiveness Research: Emerging Methods and Policy Applications (June 2010), pp. S17–S22 (6 pages)

Hughes, J. C. (2014) *How we think about dementia: Personhood, rights, ethics, the arts, and what they mean for care*. London: Jessika Kingsley Publishers.

Illeris, K. (2018) *Contemporary theories of learning* (p. 2). London: Taylor and Francis.

Institute for Healthcare Improvement (2022) *SBAR Tool: Situation- Background-Assessment-Recommendation*. [Online] maintenance. ihi.org. Available at: https://www.ihi.org/resources/pages/tools/ SBARToolkit.aspx.

Interprofessional Teamwork for Health and Social Care, Scott Reeves, Simon Lewin, Sherry Espin and Merrick Zwarenstein © 2010 Blackwell Publishing Ltd. ISBN: 978-1-405-18191-4. Promoting partnership for health Interprofessional Teamwork for Health and Social Care. Scott Reeves Simon Lewin Sherry Espin Merrick Zwarenstein. Available at: Front Matter – *Interprofessional Teamwork for Health and Social Care* – Wiley Online Library

Ioannidis, P. A. et al. (2014) 'Publication and other reporting biases in cognitive sciences: Detection, prevalence, and prevention', *Trends in Cognitive Sciences*, 18(5), pp. 235–241. Available at: https://doi.org/10.1016/j.tics.2014.02.010 (Accessed: 3 June 2022).

IPEC (2016) *Core competencies for interprofessional collaborative practice.* [Online]. Available at https://www.ipecollaborative.org/assets/2016-Update.pdf

Jeffrey, B. *et al.* (2005) *WRITING@CSU, Guide.* Available at: https://writing.colostate.edu/guides/guide.cfm?guideid=65 (Accessed: 08 August 2023).

Jelley, W., Larocque, N. and Borghese, M. (2013) 'Perceptions on the Essential Competencies for Intraprofessional Practice', *Physiotherapy Canada* 65(2), pp. 148-151. Available at: https://doi.org/10.3138%2Fptc.2012-02 (Accessed: 08 August 2023).

Johnson, O. (2019) 'General system theory and the use of process mining to improve care pathways', *Studies in Health Technology and Informatics*, 30(263), pp. 11–22. Available at: https://doi.org/10.3233/SHTI190107 (Accessed: 23 April 2022).

Jones, A. and Jones, D. (2010) 'Improving teamwork, trust and safety: An ethnographic study of an interprofessional initiative', *Journal of Interprofessional Care*, 25(3), pp. 175–181. Available at: https://doi.org/10.3109/13561820.2010.520248 (Accessed: 12 May 2022).

Jones, J. L. and Mehr, S. L. (2007) 'Foundations and assumptions of the scientist-practitioner model'. *American Behavioral Scientist*, 50(6), pp. 766–771. Available at: https://doi.org/10.1177/0002764206296454 (Accessed: 12 May 2022).

Jones, S.R. (1992). 'Was there a Hawthorne effect?'. *American Journal of Sociology*, 98(3), pp. 451–468. Available at: https://doi.org/10.1086/230046 (Accessed: 8 January 2023).

Kamper, S.J. (2020) 'Generalizability: linking evidence to practice', *Journal of Orthopaedic & Sports Physical Therapy*, 50(1), pp. 45–46. Available at: https://doi.org/10.2519/jospt.2020.0701 (Accessed: 8 January 2023).

Kemp, P., Gilding, M., Seewooruttun, K. and Walsh, H. (2016) 'A work-based learning approach for clinical support workers on mental health inpatient wards', *Nursing Standard*, 31(3), pp. 48–55. Available at: https://doi.org/10.7748/ns.2016.e10196 (Accessed: 30 October 2022).

Kim, E.J. and Seomun, G. (2020) 'Handover in Nursing: A Concept Analysis', *Research and Theory for Nursing Practice*, 34(4), pp. 297–320. Available at: https://doi.org/10.1891/rtnp-d-19-00089 (Accessed: 12 May 2022).

Kinsella, E. A. (2010) 'The art of reflective practice in health and social care: Reflections on the legacy of Donald Schön', *Reflective Practice*, 11(4), pp. 565–575. Available at: https://doi.org/10.1080/146239 43.2010.506260 (Accessed: 12 May 2022).

Kison, S. D., Moorer, K. D. and Villarosa, M. C. (2015) 'The integration of science and practice: Unique perspectives from counseling psychology students', *Counselling Psychology Quarterly*, 28(3), pp. 345–359. Available at: https://doi.org/10.1080/09515070.2015.1060193 (Accessed: 23 May 2022).

Kitto, S.C., Chesters, J. and Garbich, C. (2008) 'Quality in qualitative research', *Medical Journal of Australia*, 188(4), pp. 243–246. Available at: https://doi.org/10.5694/j.1326-5377.2008.tb01595.x (Accessed: 23 May 2022).

Kitwood, T. (1997) *Dementia reconsidered*. Berkshire: Open University Press-McGraw-Hill Education.

Knoke, D. and Yang, S. (2008) *Social network analysis*. 2nd ed. London: SAGE.

Lairumbi G. M., Molyneux, S., Snow, R. W., Marsh, K. Peshu, N. and English, M. (2008) 'Promoting the social value of research in Kenya: Examining the practical aspects of collaborative partnerships using an ethical framework', *Social Science & Medicine*, 67(5), pp. 734–747. Available at: https://doi.org/10.1016/j.socscimed.2008.02.016 (Accessed: 3 August 2022)

Lazzari, C. (1986) 'Power and conflicts in complex systems and the ethics of human relations explained by cybersystemic models', *Proceedings from the International Meeting of Cybernetic and Systems in Namur, Belgium, June 1986*. Available at: Actes – Google Books (Accessed: 4 April 2022).

Lazzari, C. (1998) *The helping relationship: How to care for others when worried about their health*. Bologna: Pitagora.

Lazzari, C. (2004) *Psychology and ethics of work and organisations*. Rome: Armando.

Lazzari, C. (2006) *Psychology and ethics of companies and business relationships*. Rome: Armando.

Lazzari, C. (2007) *How the mind works: Understanding human thoughts and behaviours*. New York: iUniverse. Amazon.

Lazzari, C. (2008) *Communication in the helping relationship*. Milan: Lampi di Stampa.

Lazzari, C. (2014) 'The assessment of attitudes during interprofessional education in psychiatry. How do mental health professionals cooperate when dealing with psychiatric patients?' *Proceedings of the International Congress of the Royal College of Psychiatrists, London, June 2014*. Available at: ResearchGate (Accessed: 4 April 2022).

Lazzari, C. (2018) 'Ethnographic and observational research in the healthcare services: Creating policies in dementia care', *Indian Journal of Medical Research and Pharmaceutical Sciences*, 5(7), pp. 8–11. Available at: https://doi.org/10.5281/zenodo.1314077 (Accessed: 5 April 2022).

Lazzari, C. (2019) 'Interprofessional education and practice, and the application of social network analysis', *CPQ Medicine* 5(4), pp. 1–12. Available at: https://doi.org/10.5281/zenodo.7393102 or https ://www.cientperiodique.com/article/CPQME/5/4 (Accessed: 8 April 2022).

Lazzari, C. (2019) 'Interprofessional Education and Practice and the Application of Social Network Analysis', *CPQ Medicine*, 5(4), pp. 1–12. Available at: ResearchGate

Lazzari, C. and Masiello, I. (2016) 'Communication neurosciences for interprofessional teams in health care', in Wrig, B. L. (ed.) *Communication skills: Challenges, importance for health care professionals and strategies for improvement*. New York: NOVA Publishers. (Accessed: 5 April 2022).

Lazzari, C. and Masiello, I. (2017a) 'Can patients differentiate when they receive integrated care by interprofessional teams? Meta-analysis of a pilot study', *European Psychiatry*, 41(S1), pp. S299–S300. Available at: https://doi.org/10.1016/j.eurpsy.2017.02.183 (Accessed: 5 April 2022).

Lazzari, C. and Masiello, I. (2017b) 'How satisfied are undergraduate students with interprofessional training? Meta-analysis of a pilot study', *European Psychiatry*, 41(S1), p. S299. Available at: https://doi.org/10.1016/j.eurpsy.2017.02.182 (Accessed: 5 April 2022).

Lazzari, C. and Masiello, I. (2017c) 'Flow experiences improve mindfulness of educational emotions during interprofessional training. Meta-analysis of a pilot study', *European Psychiatry* 41(S1), S897. Available at: https://doi.org/10.1016/j.eurpsy.2017.01.1830 (Accessed: 2 April 2022).

Lazzari, C. and Masino, M. A. (2006) *Love that heals: A guide to the helping relationships.* Milan: FrancoAngeli. University Library – Italy (Accessed: 5 April 2022).

Lazzari, C. and Masino, M. A. (2015) *Psychology and philosophy of health.* Milan: Libreriauniversitaria.it. Amazon (Accessed: 5 April 2022).

Lazzari, C. and Rabottini, M. (2021) *The assessment of interprofessional practice in psychiatry.* Kindle Books.

Lazzari, C. and Shoka, A. (2016). Chapter 2. Corporate management of patients with borderline personality disorder through integrated care, in Anderson, R. (ed.) *Borderline personality disorder (BPD): Prevalence, management options and challenges.* New York: Nova Publishers (Accessed: 5 April 2022).

Lazzari, C. and Thomas, H. (2018a) 'Concerns in dementia caregivers about threats to the personhood of patients with dementia: A narrative approach for analysis,' *Indian Journal of Medical Research and Pharmaceutical Sciences,* 5(6), pp. 20–25. Available at: ResearchGate (Accessed: 5 April 2022).

Lazzari, C. and Thomas, H. (2018b) 'Partnership in healthcare teams provides patient-centred care in dementia,' *CPQ Medicine* 1(5), pp. 1–4. Available at: ResearchGate (Accessed: 5 April 2022). Available at: https://doi.org/10.5281/zenodo.7433853 (Accessed: 5 April 2022).

Lazzari, C., Shoka, A., Papanna, B. and Mousailidis, G. (2017) 'Chapter 2. Advancing healthcare leadership: Theories of analysis and intervention in borderline personality disorder', in Columbus. A. M. (ed.) *Advances in psychology research*, Volume 131. New York: Nova Publishers.

Lazzari, C., Kotera, Y. and Thomas, H. (2019) 'Social network analysis of dementia wards in psychiatric hospitals to explore the advancement of personhood in patients with Alzheimer's disease', *Current Alzheimer Research*, 16(6), pp. 505–517. Available at: https://doi.org/10.2174/15672 05016666190612160955 (Accessed: 8 April 2022).

Lazzari, C., Kotera, Y., Green, P. and Rabottini, M. (2021) 'Social network analysis of Alzheimer's teams: A clinical review and applications in psychiatry to explore interprofessional care', *Current Alzheimer Research*, 18(5), pp. 380–398. Available at: https://doi.org/10.2174/15672 05018666210701161449 (Accessed: 4 April 2022).

Lazzari, C., Masiello, I. and Shoka, A. (2017) 'Chapter 1. Theoretical models of social mind and social thinking in interprofessional education', in Nata R. V. (ed.) *Progress in education*. Volume 48. New York: Nova Publishers.

Lazzari, C., McAleer, S. and Rabottini, M. (2022) 'The assessment of interprofessional practice in mental health nursing with ethnographic observation and social network analysis: A confirmatory and biblio-metric network study using VOSviewer', *Rivista di Psichiatria*, 57(3), pp. 115–122. Available at: https://doi.org/10.1708/3814.37989 (Accessed: 4 April 2022).

Lazzari, C., McAleer, S., Nusair, A. and Rabottini, M. (2021) 'Psychiatric training during COVID-19 pandemic benefits from integrated practice in interprofessional teams and ecological momentary e-assessment', *Rivista di Psichiatria*, 56(2), pp. 74–84. Available at: https://doi.org/10.1708/3594.35765 (Accessed: 4 April 2022).

Lazzari, C., Shoka, A. and Masiello, I. (2016) 'Chapter 3. Maladaptive behaviors in inpatients with borderline personality disorder: A behavioral game theory explanation', in Anderson, R. (ed.) *Borderline personality disorder (BPD): Prevalence, management options and challenges*. New York: Nova Publishers.

Lazzari, C., Shoka, A., Papanna, B. and Kulkarni, K. (2018) 'Current healthcare challenges in treating the borderline personality disorder "epidemic"', *British Journal of Medical Practitioners*, 11(2), p. a1112. Google Scholar

Lazzari, C., (2023). 'Theoretical Frameworks of Clinical Handovers in Healthcare Settings', *Research Highlights in Disease and Health Research Vol. 4*, pp. 125–147. Available at: ps://www.researchgate.net/publication/369688930_Handover_002

Leeman, J. and Sandelowski, M. (2012) 'Practice-based evidence and qualitative inquiry', *Journal of Nursing Scholarship* 44(2), pp. 171–179. Available at: https://doi.org/10.1111/j.1547-5069.2012.01449.x. (Accessed: 3 May 2023)

Lehna, C., Hermanns, M., Monsivais, D.B. and Engebretson, J. (2016) 'From dissertation defense to dissemination: Jump start your academic career with a scholar mentor group', *Nursing Forum* (Hillsdale), 51(1), pp. 62–69. Available at: https://doi.org/10.1111/nuf.12124 (Accessed: 3 May 2023)

Leland, N.E. (2016). 'Transitioning from defending the dissertation to dissemination: Publishing and presenting your work' [Abstract], *The Gerontologist*, 56(3), pp. 275–276. Available at: gnw162.1114.pdf (silverchair.com) (Accessed: 30 March 2023).

Lester, S. and Costley, C. (2010) 'Work-based learning at higher education level: Value, practice and critique', *Studies in Higher Education*, 35(5), pp. 561–575. Available at: https://doi.org/10.1080/03075070903216635 (Accessed: 20 June 2022).

Levac, D., Colquhoun, H. and O'Brien, K.K. (2010) 'Scoping studies: advancing the methodology', *Implementation Science*, 5(69). Available at: https://doi.org/10.1186/1748-5908-5-69 (Accessed: 20 June 2022).

Lewis, C. and Throne, R. (2021) 'Practice-based and practice-led research for dissertation development', *IGI Global*, pp. 87–107. Available at: https://www.igi-global.com/chapter/autoethnography-and-other-self-inquiry-methods-for-practice-based-doctoral-research/260930 (Accessed: 10 March 2022).

Lockhart, N. (2017) 'Social network analysis as an analytic tool for task group research: A case study of an interdisciplinary community of practice', *The Journal for Specialists in Group Work*, 42(2), pp. 152–175. Available at: http://dx.doi.org/10.1080/01933922.2017.1301610 (Accessed: 10 April 2022).

Lynas, K. and NHS Leadership Acadeour (n.d.) *Introduction to Team Development.* (Online) Available at: https://www.leadershipacadeour.nhs.uk/wp-content/uploads/2013/04/7428f23d7207f39da1eda97a dbd7bf34.pdf (Accessed: 12 April 2023).

Malthouse, R., Watts, M. and Roffey-Barensten, J. (2015) 'Reflective questions, self-questioning and managing professionally situated practice', *Research in Education*, 94, pp. 71–87. Available at: https://doi.org/10.7227%2FRIE.0024 (Accessed: 14 April 2022).

Manias, E., Bucknall, T., Woodward-Kron, R., Hughes, C., Jorm, C., Ozavci, G. and Joseph, K. (2021) 'Interprofessional and Intraprofessional Communication about Older People's Medications across Transitions of Care', *International Journal of Environmental Research and Public Health*, 18(8), p. 3925. Available at: https://doi.org/10.3390/ijerph18083925 (Accessed: 14 April 2022).

Manning, P. (1992) *Erving Goffman and modern sociology*. Stanford: Stanford University Press.

Maree, D. J. (2020) 'The applicative split: The science-practitioner model of training and practice', in Maree, D. J. (ed.) *Realism and psychological science*. Springer, Cham, pp. 43–53. Available at: https://link.springer.com/chapter/10.1007/978-3-030-45143-1_3 (Accessed: 10 April 2022).

Mathisen, V., Obstfelder, A., Lorem, G.F., and Måseide, P. (2016) 'User participation in district psychiatry. The social construction of 'users' in handovers and meetings', *Nursing Inquiry*, 23(2), pp. 169–177. Available at: https://doi.org/ 10.1111/nin.12127 (Accessed: 10 April 2022).

Maudsley, G. et al. (2018) 'A best evidence medical education (BEME) systematic review of: What works best for health professions students using mobile (hand-held) devices for educational support on clinical placements? BEME guide No. 52', *Medical Teacher*, 41(2), pp. 125–140. Available at: https://doi.org/10.1080/0142159X.2018.1508829 (Accessed: 1 May 2021).

Maxwell, T. W. (2019) 'Philosophy and practice. Why does this matter?' in Costley, C. and Fulton, J. (eds.) *Methodologies for practice research: Approaches for professional doctorates*. London: Sage.

McLeod, S. (2018) 'Maslow's Hierarchy of Needs'. [online] Canada College, Simply Psychology, p. 1. Available at: https://canadacollege.edu/dreamers/docs/Maslows-Hierarchy-of-Needs.pdf (Accessed: 11 Dec. 2023).

Mead, M. (1977) *Letters from the field: 1925–1975*. New York: Harper & Row.

Mead, M. (2004) *Studying contemporary Western society: Method and theory.* Oxford: Berghahan Books.

Melick, R. R. and Melick, S. (2010) *Teaching that transforms.* Nashville: Band H Publishing Group.

Merriam-Webster Dictionary (2021) *Meaning.* Available at: https://www.merriam-webster.com/dictionary/meaning (Accessed 24 Feb. 2022).

Merriam-Webster Dictionary (2022a) *Autoplasticity.* Available at: https://www.merriam-webster.com/dictionary/autoplasticity (Accessed: 24 Feb. 2022).

Merriam-Webster Dictionary (2022b) *Alloplasticity.* Available at: https://www.merriam-webster.com/dictionary/alloplasticity (Accessed 24 Feb. 2022).

Merriam-Webster Dictionary (2022c) *Culture.* Available at: https://www.merriam-webster.com/dictionary/culture (Accessed: 1 April 2022).

Merriam-Webster Dictionary (2019). *Definition of Communicate.* Available at: https://www.merriam-webster.com/dictionary/communicate (Accessed: 24 Feb. 2022).

Mertens, D. M. (2007) 'Transformative paradigm: Mixed methods and social justice', *Journal of Mixed Methods Research,* 1(3), pp. 212–225. Available at: https://doi/org/10.1177/1558689807302811 (Accessed: 10 April 2022).

Mertens, D. M. (2009) *Transformative research and evaluation.* New York: The Guilford Press.

Merton, R. K. (1968) *Social theory and social structure (1968 enlarged ed.).* New York: Free Press.

Mezirow, J. (2002) 'Transformative learning theory to practice', *New Directions for Adult and Continuing Education,* 1977(74), pp. 5–12. Available at: https://doi.org/10.1002/ace.7401 (Accessed: 29 March 2022).

Mezirow, J. (2003) 'Transformative learning and discourse', *Journal of Transformative Education,* 1(1), pp. 58–63. Available at: https://doi.org/10.1177/1541344603252172 (Accessed: 29 March 2022).

Miller, A. and Frederickson, N. (2006) 'Generalizable findings and idiographic problems: Struggles and successes for educational psychologists as scientist-practitioners', in Lane, D. A. and Corrie, S. (eds.) *The modern scientist-practitioner: A guide to practice in Psychology.* London: Routledge.

Montreuil, M. and Carnevale, F. (2018) 'Participatory hermeneutic ethnography: A methodological framework for health ethics research with children', *Qualitative Health Research*, 28(7), pp. 1135–1144. Available at: https:/doi.org/10.1177/1049732318757489 (Accessed: 10 April 2022).

Moreno, J. L. (1937) 'Sociometry in relation to other social sciences', *Sociometry*, 1(1/2), pp. 206–219. Available at: https://www.jstor.org/stable/2785266 (Accessed: 28 April 2022).

Moreno, L. (1941) 'Foundations of sociometry: An introduction', *Sociometry*, 4(1), pp. 15–35. Available at: https://www.jstor.org/stable/2785363 (Accessed: 28 April 2022).

Moskowitz, D. S. and Young, N. Y. (2006) 'Ecological momentary assessment: What it is and why it is a method of the future in clinical psychopharmacology', *Journal of Psychiatry Neuroscience*; 31(1), pp. 13–20. Available at: http://www.ncbi.nlm.nih.gov/pmc/articles/pmc1325062/ (Accessed: 10 April 2022).

Müller, M., Jürgens, J., Redaèlli, M., Klingberg, K., Hautz, W. E. and Stock, S. (2018) 'Impact of the communication and patient hand-off tool SBAR on patient safety: A systematic review', *BMJ Open*, 8(8), pp. e022202–e022202. Available at: https://doi.org/10.1136/bmjopen-2018-022202 (Accessed: 23 October 2022)

Murad, M.H., Asi, N., Alsawas, M. and Alahdab, F. (2016) 'New evidence pyramid', *Evidence Based Medicine* 21(4): pp. 125-127. Available at: https://doi.org/10.1136/ebmed-2016-110401 (Accessed 24 Feb. 2022).

National Health Service (Tees, Esk and Wear Valley NHS Foundation Trust) (2022) *Competency testimony North of England approvals panel.* Available at: https://www.tewv.nhs.uk/about/neap/ (Accessed: 4 April 2022).

NHS England (2014) *Interprofessional collaboration in intermediate care.* [PDF File]. Available at: https://www.england.nhs.uk/publication/making-it-happen-multi-disciplinary-team-mdt-working/

NHS Health Education England (2022) *Integrated care.* Available at: Integrated care | Health Education England (hee.nhs.uk)

Nicholls, J. R. (1984) 'An alloplastic approach to corporate culture', *International Studies of Management & Organization*, 14(4), pp. 32–63. Available at: https://doi.org/10.1080/00208825.1984.11656395 (Accessed: 3 June 2022)

Nikolopoulou, K. (2023, March 03) *What Is Generalizability? | Definition & Examples.* Scribbr. Retrieved March 20, 2023, from https://www.scribbr.com/research-bias/generalizability/

Nikolou-Walker, E. (2007) 'Critical reflections on an evaluative comparative analysis of work-based learning through organisational change mechanisms: A study of two public service organizations in Northern Ireland', *Reflective Practice* 8(4), pp. 525–543. Available at: https://doi.org/10.1080/14623940701649803 (Accessed: 3 June 2022).

Nikolou-Walker, E. (2020) 'Legal safeguarding for work-based learners in creative educational models ELDA', *Work Based Learning e-Journal,* 9(2.b), p. 55. Available at: https://wblearning-ejournal.com/uploads/text_with_images/3.eldanikolouwalkerlegalsafeguardingforworkbasedlearnersincreativeeducationalmodels1607380889.pdf (Accessed: 23 May 2022).

Nikolou-Walker, E. and Curley, H. (2011) 'Philosophical and ethical issues in Work-based learning educational research: A review of four published works', *Work-Based Learning e-Journal.* 1(2), pp. 55–79. Available at: Google (Accessed: 4 June 2022).

Nikolou-Walker, E. and Curley, H. (2012) 'An examination, evaluation and analysis of work-based learning leadership within a higher education setting', *Higher Education, Skills and Work-based Learning,* 2(2), pp. 186–200. Available at: https://eprints.mdx.ac.uk/id/eprint/16375 (Accessed: 3 June 2022).

Nikolou-Walker, E. and Garnett, J. (2004) 'Work-based learning. A new imperative: Developing reflective practice in real life', *Reflective Practice,* 5(3): pp. 297–312. Available at: https://doi.org/10.1080/1462394042000270637 (Accessed: 23 May 2022).

Nikolou-Walker, E. and Lavery, K. (2009) 'Work-based research assessment of the impact of "lean manufacturing" on health and safety education within an SME', *Research in Post-Compulsory Education,* 14(4), pp. 441–458. Available at: https://eprints.mdx.ac.uk/id/eprint/16374 (Accessed: 4 June 2022).

Nikolou-Walker, E. and Meaklim, T. (2007) 'Vocational training in higher education: A case study of work-based learning within the Police Service of Northern Ireland (PSNI)', *Research in Post-Compulsory Education,* 12(3), pp. 357–376. Available at: https://doi.org/10.1080/13596740701559829 (Accessed: 23 May 2022).

Nimmon, L. and Cristancho, S. (2019) 'When I say … networks and systems', *Medical Education*, 53(4), pp. 331–333. Available at: https://doi.org/10.1111/medu.13673 (Accessed: 28 May 2022).

Nimmon, L., Artino, A. R. and Varpio, L. (2019) 'Social network theory in interprofessional education: Revealing hidden power', *Journal of Graduate Medical Education*, 11(3), pp. 247–250. Available at: https://doi.org/10.4300%2FJGME-D-19-00253.1 (Accessed: 28 May 2022).

Northouse, P. G. (2004) *Leadership: Theory and practice.* Thousand Oaks, CA: Sage.

Nurse and Midwifery Council (2015). *The Code.* London: Nurse and Midwifery Council. Available at: https://www.nmc.org.uk/globalassets/sitedocuments/nmc-publications/nmc-code.pdf (Accessed: 15 December 2022).

Olson, R., Bidewell, J., Dune, T. and Lessey, N. (2016) 'Developing cultural competence through self-reflection in interprofessional education: Findings from an Australian university', *Journal of Interprofessional Care*, 30(3), pp. 347–354. Available at: https://doi/org/10.3109/13561820.2016.1144583 (Accessed: 10 September 2022).

Overholser, J. C. (1993) 'Elements of the Socratic method: I. Systematic questioning', *Psychotherapy: Theory, Research, Practice, Training*, 30(1), p. 67. Available at: https://psycnet.apa.org/doi/10.1037/0033-3204.30.1.67 (Accessed: 29 March 2022).

Passini, S. (2010) 'Moral reasoning in a multicultural society: Moral inclusion and moral exclusion', *Journal for the Theory of Social Behaviour*, 40, p. 4. Available at: https://doi.org/10.1111/j.1468-5914.2010.00440.x (Accessed: 29 March 2022).

Perry, W. G. (1970) *Forms of intellectual and ethical development in the college years: A scheme.* London: Holt, Rinehart and Winston.

Persson, A. (2018) *Framing Social Interaction: Continuities and Cracks in Goffman's Frame Analysis.* First ed. Boca Raton, FL: Taylor & Francis, 2018.

Peters, D. H. et al. (2013) 'Implementation research: What it is and how to do it', *BMJ*, 347, p. f6753. Available at: https://doi.org/10.1136/bmj.f6753 (Accessed: 24 February 2022).

Polit, D. F. and Beck, C. T. (2022) *Essentials of nursing research*, 10th edition. London: Wolters Kluver.

Polit, D.F. and Beck, C.T. (2010) 'Generalisation in quantitative and qualitative research: Ourths and strategies,' *International Journal of Nursing Studies*, 47(11), pp. 1451–1458. Available at: https://doi. org/10.1016/j.ijnurstu.2010.06.004 (Accessed: 24 February 2022).

Ponterotto, J.G. (2006). 'Brief note on the origins, evolution, and meaning of the qualitative research concept thick description', *The Qualitative Report*, 11(3), pp. 538–549. Available at: http://www.nova.edu/ssss/ QR/QR11-3/ponterotto.pdf (Accessed: 24 February 2022).

Poulos, C. (2021) *Essentials of autoethnography*. Washington: American Psychological Association.

Prell, C. (2012) *Social network analysis: History, theory and methodology*. London: Sage.

Prentice, D., Engel, J., Taplay, K. and Stobbe, K. (2015) 'Interprofessional Collaboration: The Experience of Nursing and Medical Students' Interprofessional Education. *Global Qualitative Nursing Research*, 2: p. 2333393614560566. Available at: https://doi. org/10.1177/2333393614560566 (Accessed: 24 February 2022).

Reeves, S. and Lewin S. (2004) 'Interprofessional collaboration in the hospital: strategies and meanings', *Journal of Health Services Research & Policy*, 9(4), pp. 218–225. Available at: https://doi. org/10.1258/1355819042250140 (Accessed: 24 February 2022).

Reeves, S. (2003) 'A systematic review of the effects of interprofessional education on staff involved in the care of adults with mental health problems', *Journal of Psychiatric and Mental Health Nursing*, 8(6), pp. 533–542. Available at: https://doi.org/10.1046/j.1351-0126.2001.00420.x (Accessed: 24 February 2022).

Reeves, S. and Freeth, D. (2006) 'Re-examining the evaluation of interprofessional education for community mental health teams with a different lens: Understanding presage, process and product factors', *Journal of Psychiatric and Mental Health Nursing*, 13(6), pp. 765–770. Available at: https://doi.org/10.1111/j.1365-2850.2006.01032.x (Accessed: 5 June 2022).

Reeves, S. et al. (2011) 'A scoping review to improve conceptual clarity of interprofessional interventions', *Journal of Interprofessional Care*, 25(3), pp. 167–174. Available at: https://doi.org/10.3109/13561820.2010.529960 (Accessed: 5 June 2022).

Reeves, S. et al. (2013) 'Interprofessional education: Effects on professional practice and healthcare outcomes (update)', *Cochrane Database Systematic Reviews*, 3(CD002213). Available at: https://doi.org/10.1002/14651858.CD002213.pub3 (Accessed: 29 March 2022).

Reeves, S., Pelone, F., Harrison, R., Goldman, J. and Zwarenstein, M. (2017) 'Interprofessional collaboration to improve professional practice and healthcare outcomes', *The Cochrane Database of Systematic Reviews*, 6(6), CD000072. Available at: https://doi.org/10.1002/14651858.CD000072.pub3 (Accessed: 4 April 2022).

Reeves, S., Xyrichis, A., Zwarenstein, M. (2018) 'Teamwork, collaboration, coordination, and networking: Why we need to distinguish between different types of interprofessional practice', *Journal of Interprofessional Care*, 32(1), pp. 1–3. Available at: https://doi.org/10.1080/13561820.2017.1400150 (Accessed: 10 April 2022).

Reuters (2003). *Advertising Solutions.* [webpage]. Available at: https://www.reutersagency.com/en/who-we-serve/professionals/ (Accessed: 29 March 2023).

Rhydderch, M., Elwyn, G., Marshall, M. and Grol, R. (2004) 'Organisational change theory and the use of indicators in general practice', *BMJ Quality and Safety*, 13(3), pp. 213–217. Available at: https://doi.org/10.1136/qhc.13.3.213 (Accessed: 23 May 2022)

Rickard, F., Lu, F., Gustafsson, L., MacArthur, C., Cummins, C., Coker, I., Wilson, A., Mane, K., Manneh, K., Manaseki-Holland, S. (2022) 'Clinical handover communication at maternity shift changes and women's safety in Banjul, the Gambia: A mixed-methods study.' *BMC Pregnancy and Childbirth*, (22)1, p. 21. Available at: https://doi.org/10.1186/s12884-022-05052-9 (Accessed: 24 February 2022).

Roy, C. (2014) *Generating middle-range theory: From evidence to practice.* New York: Springer Publishing Company.

Royal College of Nursing (2022) *Teamwork.* Available at: https://www.rcn.org.uk/clinical-topics/Patient-safety-and-human-factors/Professional-Resources/Teamwork (Accessed: 5 June 2022).

Royal College of Psychiatrists (2019) *Working Well Together: Evidence and Tools to Enable Co-production in Mental Health Commissioning.* London: National Collaborating Centre for Mental Health. Available at: https://www.rcpsych.ac.uk/improving-care/nccmh/service-design-and-development/working-well-together (Accessed: 15 December 2022).

Royal College of Surgeons England (2022) *Professional Code of Conduct.* London: Royal College of Surgeons. Available at: https://www. rcseng.ac.uk/standards-and-research/standards-and-guidance/service-standards/surgical-care-team-guidance/professional-code-of-conduct/ (Accessed: 15 December 2022).

Saldaña, J. (2011) *Fundamentals of qualitative research.* Oxford, England: Oxford University Press.

Schermuly, C. C. and Meyer, B. (2020) 'Transformational leadership, psychological empowerment, and flow at work', *European Journal of Work and Organisational Psychology,* 29(5), pp. 740–752. Available at: https://doi.org/10.1080/1359432X.2020.174905 (Accessed: 4 May 2022).

Schmidt, M. (2010) 'Learning from teaching experience: Dewey's theory and preservice teachers' learning', *Journal of Research in Music Education,* 58(2), pp. 131–146. Available at: https://doi. org/10.1177/0024429410368723 (Accessed: 10 April 2022).

Schön, D. A. (1987) *Educating the reflective practitioner: Toward a new design for teaching and learning in the professions.* Jossey-Bass higher education series. San Francisco, CA: Jossey-Bass.

Schön, D. A. (1991) *The reflective practitioner: How professionals think in action.* London: Routledge.

Schön, D. A. and Rein, M. (1994) *Frame reflection.* New York: Basic Books.

Sentra, J. (2017) *Social network analysis, 4th ed.* London: Sage.

Shapiro, D. (2002) 'Renewing the scientist-practitioner model', *Psychologist-Leicester,* 15(5), pp. 232–235. Available at: Renewing the scientist-practitioner model | The Psychologist (bps.org.uk) (Accessed: 1 June 2022)

Shiffman, S., Stone, A. A. and Hufford, M. R. (2008) 'Ecological momentary assessment', *Annual Review of Clinical Psychology,* 40(1), pp. 328–341. Available at: https://doi.org/10.3758/brm.40.1.328 (Accessed: 4 May 2022)

Shoham, D. A., Harris, J. K., Mundt, M. and McGaghie, W. (2016) 'A network model of communication in an interprofessional team of healthcare professionals: A cross-sectional study of a burn unit', *Journal of Interprofessional Care,* 30(5), pp. 661–667. Available at: https://doi.org/10.1080/13561820.2016.1203296 (Accessed: 4 May 2022)

Siebert, S. and Costley, C. (2013) 'Conflicting values in reflection on professional practice', *Higher Education, Skills and Work-Based Learning*, 3(3), pp. 156–167. Available at: https://doi.org/10.1108/HESWBL-07-2011-0032 (Accessed: 28 September 2022).

Slamecka, V. (2022) 'Meaning of information'. *Encyclopaedia Britannica*. https://www.britannica.com/technology/information-processing (Accessed: 4 May 2022).

Smaldone, A. *et al.* (2019) 'Dissemination of PhD dissertation research by dissertation format: A retrospective cohort study,' *Journal of Nursing Scholarship*, 51(5), pp. 599–607. Available at: https://doi.org/10.1111/jnu.12504 (Accessed: 30 March 2023).

Smeulers, M., Lucas, C. and Vermeulen, H. (2014) 'What is the best nursing handover style to ensure continuity of information for hospital patients?' [Internet] [cited 2022Dec23]. Available from: https://www.cochrane.org/CD009979/EPOC_what-best-nursing-handover-style-ensure-continuity-information-hospital-patients

Stone, A. (2007) *The science of real-time data capture*. Oxford: Oxford University Press.

Stone, A. and Shiffman, S. (1994) 'Ecological momentary assessment (Ema) in behavioral medicine', *Annals of Behavioral Medicine*, 16(3), pp. 199–202. Available at: https://doi.org/10.1093/abm/16.3.199 (Accessed: 10 May 2022).

Swanwick, T. (ed.) (2010) *Understanding medical education*. Oxford: Wiley-Blackwell.

Swanwick, T. and McKimm, J. (2010) 'What is clinical leadership … and why is it important?' *The Clinical Teacher*, 8(1), pp. 22–26. Available at: https://doi.org/10.1111/j.1743-498X.2010.00423.x (Accessed: 10 May 2022).

Tan, H.C., Ho, J.A., Kumarusamy, R. and Sambasivan, M. (2021) 'Measuring social desirability bias: Do the full and short versions of the Marlowe-Crowne Social Desirability scale matter?,' *Journal of Empirical Research on Human Research Ethics*, p.155626462110460. Availble at: doi:https://doi.org/10.1177/15562646211046091 (Accessed: 10 May 2022).

Tarling, J. (2016) 'Could flow psychology change the way we think about vocational learning and stem the tide of poor wellbeing affecting our students? Ask the students, they'll tell you', *Research in Post-Compulsory Education*, 21(3), pp. 302–305. Available at: https://doi.org/10.1080/13596748.2016.1195171 (Accessed: 10 May 2022).

Taylor, D. C. M. and Hamdy, H. (2013) 'Adult learning theories: Implications for learning and teaching in medical education: AMEE Guide No. 83', *Medical Teacher*, 35(11), pp. e1561–e1572. Available at: https://doi.org/10.3109/0142159X.2013.828153 (Accessed: 10 May 2022).

The Farlex Free Dictionary. [Online]. *Definition of 'Interprofessional'.* Available at: https://medical-dictionary.thefreedictionary.com/intraprofessional+team

The Joint Commission. Patient Safety [Internet]. *The Joint Commission.* [cited 2023Feb6]. Available from: https://www.jointcommission.org/resources/patient-safety

Thistlethwaite, J. (2012) 'Interprofessional education: A review of context, learning and the research agenda', *Medical Education*, 46(1), pp. 58–70. Available at: https://doi.org/10.1111/j.1365-2923.2011.04143.x (Accessed: 3 February 2022).

Thistlethwaite, J., Moran, M. and World Health Organization Study Group on Interprofessional Education and Collaborative Practice (2010) 'Learning outcomes for interprofessional education (IPE): Literature review and synthesis', *Journal of Interprofessional Care*, 24(5), pp. 503–513. Available at: https://doi.org/10.3109/13561820.2010.483366 (Accessed: 3 February 2022).

Thompson, S. and Thompson, N. (2018) *The critically reflective practitioner.* London: Macmillan Education UK.

Tomlin, G., and Borgetto, B. (2011) 'Research Pyramid: A New Evidence-based Practice Model for Occupational Therapy', *The American Journal of Occupational Therapy*, 65(2), pp. 189–196. Available at: https://doi.org/10.5014/ajot.2011.000828 (Accessed: 3 February 2022).

Tsvetovat, M. and Kouznetosov A. (2011) *Social network analysis for startups.* Sebastopol, CA: O'Reilly.

Umberfield, E., Ghaferi, A.A., Krein, S.L. and Manojlovich, M. (2019) 'Using Incident Reports to Assess Communication Failures and Patient Outcomes', *The Joint Commission Journal on Quality and Patient Safety*, 45(6), pp. 406–413. Available at: doi:https://doi.org/10.1016/j.jcjq.2019.02.006. (Accessed: 3 February 2022).

van Diggele, C., Roberts, C., Burgess, A. and Mellis, C. (2020) 'Interprofessional education: Tips for design and implementation', *BMC Medical Education*, 20(S2). Available at: 10.1186/s12909-020-02286-z (Accessed: 10 September 2022).

van Eck N. J. and Waltman L. (2017) 'Citation-based clustering of publications using CitNetExplorer and VOSviewer', *Scientometrics* 111(2), pp. 1053–1070. Available at: https://doi.org/10.1007/s11192-017-2300-7 (Accessed: 23 April 2022).

van Eck, N. J. and Waltman, L. (2010) 'Software survey: VOSviewer, a computer program for bibliometric mapping', *Scientometrics*, 84(2), pp. 523–538. Available at: https://doi.org/10.1007/s11192-009-0146-3 (Accessed: 23 April 2022).

van Manen, M. (2015) *Pedagogical tact: Knowing what to do when you don't know what to do.* London: Routledge.

van Manen, M. (2016) *Phenomenology of practice.* (2nd ed.) New York: Routledge.

Von Bertalanffy, L. (1968) 'The meaning of general system theory', in von Bertalanffy, *General system theory: Foundations, development, applications.* New York: George Braziller, pp. 30–53.

Von Bertalanffy, L. (1969) *General system theory.* Revised edition. New York: George Braziller.

Von Bertallanfy, L. (1972) 'The history and status of general system theory', *The Acadeour of Management Journal*, 15(4), pp. 407–426.

Wainrib, S. (2005) 'Autoplastic', in de Mijolla, A. (ed.) *International dictionary of psychoanalysis* (Vol. 1). USA: Gale eBooks, p. 144. Available at: https://psycnet.apa.org/record/2005-15637-000 (Accessed 24 Feb. 2022).

Walsh, C.L., Gordon, M.F., Marshall. M., Wilson, F. and Hunt, T. (2005) 'Interprofessional capability: A developing framework for interprofessional education', *Nurse Education and Practice*, 5(4), pp. 230–237. Available at: https://doi.org/10.1016/j.nepr.2004.12.004 (Accessed 24 Feb. 2022).

Waltman, L., van Eck, N. and Noyons, E. (2010) 'A unified approach to mapping and clustering of bibliometric networks', *Journal of Infometrics*, 4(4), pp. 629–635. Available at: https://doi.org/10.1016/j.joi.2010.07.002 (Accessed: 29 March 2022).

Wang, S., Moss, J.R., Hiller, J.E. (2006) 'Applicability and transferability of interventions in evidence-based public health', *Health Promotion International*, 21, pp. 76–83. Available at: https://doi.org/10.1093/heapro/dai025 (Accessed: 29 March 2022).

Wasserman, S. and Faust, K. (1994) *Social network analysis: Methods and applications*. Cambridge: Cambridge University Press.

Watzlawick, P., Bevelas, J. B. and Jackson, D. D. (1967) *Pragmatic of human communication*. London: W. W. Norton and Company.

Way, D., Jones, L. and Bushing, N. (2000) 'Implementation strategies: Collaboration in primary care–Family doctors & nurse practitioners delivering shared care', *Toronto: The Ontario College of Family Physicians*. Available at: http://www.ocfp.on. ca/english/ocfp/communications/publications/default.asp?s¼41

West, M. A. and Farr, J. L. (eds.) (1990) *Innovation and creativity at work: Psychological and organizational strategies*. Chichester, England: John Wiley & Sons.

WHO [World Health Organization]. *Communicating during patients handovers*. WHO. 2007. [Internet] [cited 2022Dec23]. Available at: https://cdn.who.int/media/docs/default-source/patient-safety/patient-safety-solutions/ps-solution3-communication-during-patient-handovers.pdf

Wiener, N. (1954) *The human use of human beings: Cybernetics and society*. London: Da Capo Press.

Wiener, N. (2013) *Cybernetics*. Boston: The MIT Press.

Wiener, N. (2019) *Cybernetics of control and communication in the animal and machine*. Boston: The MIT Press.

Willet, L., Houston, T. K., Heudebert, G. R. and Estrada, C. (2012) 'Use of ecological momentary assessment to determine which structural factors impact perceived teaching quality of attending rounds', *Journal of Graduate Medical Education*, 4(3), pp. 322–328. Available at: https://doi.org/10.4300/JGME-D-11-00265.1 (Accessed: 22 April 2022).

World Health Organization [WHO] (2010). *Framework for action on interprofessional education and collaborative practice*. Genève, Switzerland: World Health Organization. Available at: https://www.who.int/publications/i/item/framework-for-action-on-interprofessional-education-collaborative-practice (Accessed: 3 February 2022).

Yang, S., Keller, F. B. and Zheng, L. (2016) *Social network analysis: Methods and examples*. London: Sage Publications.

Yanow, D. (2018) *Evidence-based policy. Encyclopaedia Britannica*. Available at: https://www.britannica.com/topic/evidence-based-policy (Accessed: 3 April 2022).

Yoshiuchi, K., Yamamoto, Y. and Akabayashi, A. (2008) 'Application of ecological momentary assessment in stress-related diseases', *Biopsychosocial Medicine* 2(13), pp. 1–6. Available at: https://doi.org/10.1186/1751-0759-2-13 (Accessed: 3 April 2022).

Zwarenstein, M. and Reeves, S. (2006) 'Knowledge translation and interprofessional collaboration: Where the rubber of evidence-based care hits the road of teamwork', *Journal of Continuing Education in the Health Professions*, 26(1), pp. 46–54. Available at: https://doi.org/10.1002/chp.50 (Accessed: 5 February 2022).

Biographies

Carlo Lazzari MD

Carlo Lazzari is a medical graduate with interest in interprofessional practice, interdisciplinary handovers, and teamwork in healthcare organisations. He has published extensively on these topics and developed new methods to assess collaborative practice in healthcare while formulating theories and policies for better cooperative healthcare organisations. He has published on work and organisational psychology, interprofessional practice, work conflicts and corporate policies.

Carol Costley PhD M.A. B.Ed. Cert. Ed.

Prof Carol Costley is a Professor of Work and Learning at Middlesex University, London. She holds a Master's Degree in Work Based Learning Studies and also holds professional qualifications in teaching and learning. Prof Costley works with organisations in the private, public, community and voluntary sectors internationally in the learning and teaching of work-based, taught and research degrees. She is Chair of the International Conference on Professional Doctorates 2009- present, Chair of the 'Association of Practice Doctorates' 2009- present and 'Researching Work and Learning' conference series committee member 1999- present. She has published extensively in these topics.

Elda Nikolou-Walker EdD

Dr Elda-Nikolou Walker is Senior Lecturer at Middlesex University, London. Her research interest focuses on work-based and tacit organisational learning, including self-reflective practice and ethnographic/ autoethnographic research. She has collaborated in this study with her experience in corporate education and advancing organisational culture by addressing gaps in training, improving self-reflective practice, ethnographic research methods, and ad-hoc educational programs. Dr Nikolou-Walker advocates for practice-based evidence as a route to evidence in private and public organisational sectors.

www.ingramcontent.com/pod-product-compliance
Lightning Source LLC
Chambersburg PA
CBHW031854200326
41597CB00012B/402